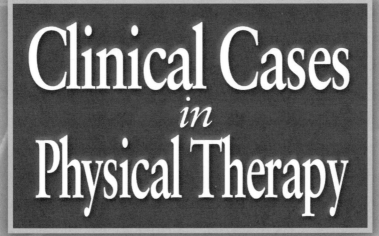

Clinical Cases
in
Physical Therapy

To Leslee, Jeanne, Eric, Christopher, Katie, and Michael, whose love, patience, and understanding made this contribution possible

Contributors

Michael B. Ashley, PT
Ashley & Kuzma Physical Therapy and
    Photomedicine
Erie, Pennsylvania

Angela M. Baeten, PT
Consultant
Abrams, Wisconsin

Amy Tremback-Ball, MSPT
Assistant Professor, Physical Therapy
    Department
College Misericordia
Dallas, Pennsylvania

Allison T. Behm, MSPT
Staff Physical Therapist
Mercy Hospital
Scranton, Pennsylvania

Marybeth Grant Beuttler, PT, MS
Assistant Professor, Physical Therapy
    Department
University of Scranton
Scranton, Pennsylvania

Donna Bowers, PT, MPH, PCS
Instructor, Department of Physical Therapy
    & Human Movement Science
Sacred Heart University
Fairfield, Connecticut

Nicole A. Boyle, MSPT
Binghamton, New York

Trista L. Bratlee, MSPT
Pittston, Pennsylvania

Mark A. Brimer, PT, PhD
Administrator, Orthopaedics
Holmes Regional Medical Center
Melbourne, Florida

Laurie Brogan, MSPT
Staff Physical Therapist
Sports Injury Treatment Center
Scranton, Pennsylvania

Kathleen M. Buccieri, PT, MS, PCS
Clinical Education Director, Physical Therapy
    Department
Ithaca College at University of Rochester
    Campus
Rochester, New York

Christopher R. Chelius, Jr., MSPT
Lead Physical Therapist and Center
    Coordinator of Clinical Education
Manatawny Manor Nursing and Rehabilitation
    Center
Pottstown, Pennsylvania

Stacia M. Ciak, MSPT
Hunlock Creek, Pennsylvania

Jason A. Craig, MCSP, DPhil
Assistant Professor, Physical Therapy
    Department
Marymount University (Ballston Campus)
Arlington, Virginia

Kristina A. Dillon, MSPT
Binghamton, New York

Carolyn J. Engdahl, MSPT
Mountain Top, Pennsylvania

Andrea Falcone, MSPT
Pediatric Physical Therapist with HFM
    BOCES
Johnstown, New York

Renee M. Hakim, PT, PhD, NCS
Assistant Professor, Physical Therapy
  Department
University of Scranton
Scranton, Pennsylvania

Jennifer Holmes, MSPT
Staff Physical Therapist
Massapequa Pain Management and
  Rehabilitation
Massapequa, Long Island, New York

Rett Holmes, MSPT
Senior Staff Physical Therapist
Physical Therapy Plus
Washington, New Jersey

Thomas Hudson, MS, PT, PCS
Assistant Professor, Physical Therapy
  Department
Consultant, Gannon University and Erie
  Homes for Children and Adults
Erie, Pennsylvania

Marianne Janssen, PT, EdD, ATC
Director of Clinical Education
Department of Physical Therapy Education
Elon University
Elon, North Carolina

Timothy L. Kauffman, PT, PhD
Kauffman-Gamber Physical Therapy
Lancaster, Pennsylvania

Edmund M. Kosmahl, PT, EdD
Professor, Physical Therapy Department
University of Scranton
Scranton, Pennsylvania

Nicholas J Kuharcik, MSPT
Larksville, Pennsylvania

MaryAlice Lachman, MSPT
Staff Physical Therapist
NovaCare Rehabilitation
Collegeville, Pennsylvania

Amy S. Lambert, MSPT
Lake Ariel, Pennsylvania

Kevin J. Lawrence, PT, MS, OCS
Assistant Professor, Physical Therapy
  Department
College Misericordia
Dallas, Pennsylvania

Holly Leaman, MSPT
Staff Physical Therapist
Maryview Rehabilitation Hospital
Portsmouth, Virginia

Beatriz Lizaso, MSPT
Pembroke Pines, Florida

Mark V. Lombardi, MSPT, MA, ATC
Sports Injury Treatment Center
Scranton, Pennsylvania

Michelle M. Lusardi, PT, PhD
Associate Professor, Department of Physical
  Therapy and Human Movement Science
Sacred Heart University
Fairfield, Connecticut

Diane E. Madras, PT, PhD
Assistant Professor, Physical Therapy
  Department
College Misericordia
Dallas, Pennsylvania

Robert Marsico, PT, EdD
Adjunct Assistant Professor, Physical Therapy
  Department
Richard Stockton College of New Jersey
Pomona, New Jersey

Colleen Medlin, MSPT
Physical Therapist
HealthSouth Spine Center of Baltimore
Baltimore, Maryland

Keith Meyer, CP
Director, Prosthetic Services
Keystone Prosthetics and Orthotics Inc.
Clarks Summit, Pennsylvania

Gerri M. Misunas, MSPT
Staff Physical Therapist
Sports Injury Treatment Center
Scranton, Pennsylvania

Georganne N. Molnar, MSPT
Newport, Pennsylvania

Kelley A. Moran, MSPT, DPT, ATC, CSCS
Associate Professor, Physical Therapy
    Department
College Misericordia
Dallas, Pennsylvania

Michael Moran, PT, ScD
Professor, Physical Therapy Department
College Misericordia
Dallas, Pennsylvania

Kristin E. Murray, MSPT
Pediatric Physical Therapist
Archway Programs Early Intervention
Atco, New Jersey

Karen W. Nolan, PT, MS, PCS
Assistant Professor, Physical Therapy
    Department
Ithaca College at University of Rochester
    Campus
Rochester, New York

Patricia O'Shea, MSPT
Long Valley, New Jersey

Maureen Romanow Pascal, PT, MS, NCS
Assistant Professor, Physical Therapy
    Department
College Misericordia
Dallas, Pennsylvania

David Patrick, MSPT, CPO
Director, Orthotic Services
Keystone Prosthetics and Orthotics Inc.
Clarks Summit, Pennsylvania

Steven D. Pheasant, PT, PhD
Assistant Professor, Physical Therapy
    Department
College Misericordia
Dallas, Pennsylvania

Kristen R. Pizzano, MSPT
Exeter, Pennsylvania

Pamela J. Reynolds, PT, EdD
Associate Professor, Physical Therapy
    Department
Gannon University
Erie, Pennsylvania

Jonathan Sakowski, MSPT
Adjunct Assistant Professor, Physical
    Therapy Department
College Misericordia
Dallas, Pennsylvania

John Sanko, PT, EdD
Associate Professor, Physical Therapy
    Department
University of Scranton
Scranton, Pennsylvania

Dawn M. Schaeffer, MSPT
Perkasie, Pennsylvania

Eric Shamus, PT, PhD, CSCS
Assistant Professor, College of Osteopathic
    Medicine
Nova Southeastern University
Fort Lauderdale, Florida

Jennifer Shamus, PT, PhD, CSCS
Clinical Specialist, Administrator
Healthsouth Sports Medicine
Pembroke Pines, Florida

Colleen Kimberly Smith, MSPT
Saylorsburg, Pennsylvania

Melissa A. Strohl, MSPT
Lehighton, Pennsylvania

Amy L. Szumski, MSPT
Scranton, Pennsylvania

Gary Tomalis, MSPT
Wilkes-Barre, Pennsylvania

Barbara Reddien Wagner, PT, MHA
Academic Coordinator of Clinical Education
University of Scranton
Scranton, Pennsylvania

John Wojnarski, MSPT
Dallas, Pennsylvania

Loraine D. Zelna, MSRT (R)(MR)(ARRT)
Associate Professor/Clinical Coordinator,
    Medical Imaging Department
College Misericordia
Dallas, Pennsylvania

With the first edition of *Clinical Cases in Physical Therapy*, Mark Brimer and Mike Moran set the standard for using clinical situations to exemplify the best aspects of our practice. These cases illustrated how each patient must be approached thoughtfully, and how expert clinical decisions must be applied in each patient situation. This text likewise "puts a face" on physical therapist education and practice. As students and clinicians, we are inundated with facts, concepts, and theories, often to the point that we begin to lose sight of what drew us to this profession in the first place. Descriptions of clinical cases remind us that we deal with people, and that all our knowledge and skill must ultimately be used to affect the life and welfare of a single individual.

Continuing the tradition established in the first edition, the second edition of *Clinical Cases in Physical Therapy* makes excellent use of cases as a teaching tool. We are again able to see how experienced clinicians examine, evaluate, and intervene in specific situations. To enhance pedagogy, learning objectives have been added to the beginning of each case. References to the peer-reviewed literature have likewise been included in these cases. These references direct readers to additional information on each topic and underscore the need to draw upon the growing body of knowledge that provides evidence for our decisions. The second edition also extends the use of case studies to encompass diverse aspects of physical therapist practice. We are now given insight into how physical therapists might react to situations that do not directly involve patient care, but situations that are nonetheless resolved successfully with skill, knowledge, and expertise. For example, cases are used to illustrate how therapists manage issues related to documentation, clinical edu-

cation, ethics, as well as many other areas related to physical therapist practice.

Hence, the second edition of *Clinical Cases in Physical Therapy* has evolved to demonstrate how cases reflect the depth and scope of our practice. Moreover, these cases are now organized according to the practice patterns and elements of management established in the *Guide to Physical Therapist Practice*, second edition. Rather than turning these cases into a fixed template or cookbook, this effort to organize and analyze according to the *Guide* helps point the way through each case in a logical and effective manner. The structure and organization of the second edition of *Clinical Cases in Physical Therapy* represent an outstanding effort by Brimer and Moran to unite our profession and provide us with a common language and strategy for examining the way we practice.

As physical therapists, we now recognize that case reports serve a vital role in our profession. We must be comfortable with the idea that clinical cases do not just document unusual patients, but that cases represent the primary way that we communicate and teach one another about the various aspects of our practice. *Clinical Cases in Physical Therapy*, 2nd edition, fulfills a vital role in classroom and clinical settings because it offers a compendium of knowledge about our profession. It is rare that a single text can be applicable to all aspects of a profession as diverse as physical therapy, but Brimer and Moran and their contributors offer some genuine pearls of wisdom to every reader. Once again, *Clinical Cases in Physical Therapy* shows us that each patient or clinical situation requires our thoughtful and skilled approach, and this idea has been, and always will be, the cornerstone of our profession.

Charles D. Ciccone, PT, PhD

Preface

The profession of physical therapy has undergone significant growth and development since the first edition of *Clinical Cases in Physical Therapy* was published almost 10 years ago. Since then, the profession has made great strides in developing and implementing the *Guide to Physical Therapist Practice*, 2nd edition, the foundation for describing and implementing physical therapy clinical practice. The goal of this text is to build upon the concepts presented in the *Guide to Physical Therapist Practice*, 2nd edition, and provide real-life examples of how therapists can use the *Guide* for patient care opportunities.

Each case in *Clinical Cases in Physical Therapy*, 2nd edition, begins with learning objectives designed to assist the reader in examining the multiple intricacies of clinical practice. Similar to the *Guide, Clinical Cases in Physical Therapy*, 2nd edition, focuses upon enhancement of quality of care, promotion of appropriate utilization of services, recognition of variations in clinical practice, the importance of sound documentation, and the value of professional ethics. Throughout each case the reader is provided with questions designed to stimulate further investigation and enhance clinical decision making. Patient care outcomes are provided for most cases. The outcomes serve to demonstrate how patient care issues were brought to closure. Peer-reviewed and other references are provided at the end of each case.

Cases have been carefully organized according to practice patterns and elements of care management. Attention was given to avoiding a "cookie-cutter" case presentation so that variations of clinical analysis and approaches can be used by the reader to find the best patient care outcome. This includes encouraging the reader to evaluate the efficacy of intervention provided and determine if it aligns with the clinical and functional goals presented.

To provide a methodology for analysis and learning, a matrix has been included at the end of the text. The matrix contains groupings under which specific practice patterns can be examined. As the reader will note, the cases are also ordered by level of complexity to allow progression of learning opportunities. Additionally, several cases have the distinction of being included in more than one practice pattern, thereby reflecting the complexity of actual patient care opportunities frequently encountered in the clinical setting.

More than anything else, *Clinical Cases in Physical Therapy*, 2nd edition, furthers understanding of the complex role the profession has in assimilating all patient care information with skill, knowledge, and expertise. The cases have been designed to provide a conceptual framework for understanding how practice patterns can be used to enhance the delivery of quality health care services.

Mark A. Brimer
Michael L. Moran

Acknowledgments

In any complex endeavor, many individuals lend varying forms of assistance. We thank all of them. We would like to specifically thank the library staff at College Misericordia for their tireless and good-natured help. Also, our thanks go to Chuck Ciccone for his support over the years and for writing the foreword to both editions. Finally, we gratefully thank Katie Moran for her sense of humor and editorial skills.

Contents

LEARNING OBJECTIVES

The reader will be able to:

1. Describe how the physical therapy examination process is important in establishing patient-centered goals and outcomes.

2. Identify how deficiencies in documentation can affect communication and result in inefficient care.

The reader should know that the patient was entering his fifth week of physical therapy intervention when he was added to the caseload.

Examination

HISTORY

The patient was a 94-year-old male who lived independently at home before sustaining a fall that resulted in a displaced C-1 fracture. The initial physician's order was for "PT eval and treat per plan of care." The patient was retired, and his son was the primary contact. The physician documented that a cervical collar was in place, that the patient reported persistent neck and left knee pain, and that the patient had full use of all extremities. Knee crepitus was recorded and documented as osteoarthritis. Medications included Procardia, Relafen, Darvocet, and Hytrin. Librium (25 mg t.i.d.) was discontinued. Nursing reported patient complaints of neck pain and noncompliance with the cervical collar. The assistance of two persons was needed to transfer the patient to a bedside chair, and the patient's tolerance for sitting was 10 minutes.

Based on the medical record review of admission information, what data might be expected in the physical therapy documentation after further history review, the systems review, and the tests and measures portion of the examination are completed?

The *Guide to Physical Therapist Practice* (p. 42)[1] defines patient history as "from both the past and the present." Therefore, one can expect such information as the patient's level of education, history of therapy intervention, living environment (e.g., devices, environmental barriers), medical history, and functional status/activity level. It would also be reasonable to expect data on communication ability as well as on cardiovascular/pulmonary, musculoskeletal, and neuromuscular systems. Tests and measures might provide baseline data in such areas as cognition, pain ratings, range of motion (especially the left knee), strength, positioning, bed mobility, endurance, transfers, balance, and gait.

The Initial Examination Documentation

The following was a summary of the documentation provided in the medical record by the examining physical therapist:

The patient was a 94-year-old male who lived alone in a two-bedroom home. He was using a cane for ambulation when his left knee buckled and he fell. He was found injured by his county home health aide. The patient was diagnosed with a displaced fracture of C-1. A cervical collar was in place. He exhibited functional mobility of all extremities except that bilateral shoulder joint flexion and abduction was limited to 100 degrees and his left knee lacked 15 degrees of extension. He exhibited fair left quad strength within his active range. General strength was fair to good. He transferred from bed to chair with a flexed posture and with moderate assistance of one.

Goals: Short-term—

1. Minimally assisted transfers.

2. Independent ambulation with assistive device to be determined.
Goals: Long-term—(blank)
Rehabilitation potential—(blank)
Plan of care: 5×/week for gait training, general strengthening, transfer training, and left knee rehabilitation.

Discussion of the Initial Examination Findings

The examining therapist did not address all of the expected examination areas. Some helpful information, such as that the patient used a cane and lived in a two-bedroom home, was obtained. However, many questions were unasked, including whether there were any environmental barriers, why home health care was received, and what the patient's prior functional level was.

The systems review portion of the examination lacked baseline cardiovascular/pulmonary system data and provided only minimal musculoskeletal system data pertaining to range-of-motion measurements and strength grades. The patient's tolerance for activity was only minimally defined, and there was no documentation of pain or positioning. Transfers were briefly addressed; however, gait and bed mobility were not assessed. It would be reasonable to expect such data or an explanation as to why they were not obtained.

Despite the limited examination data available, the therapist established two goals. The ambulation goal presented appears to be a long-term goal, not a short-term goal, and lacks validity because baseline data are lacking. The transfer goal lacks a time frame for achievement. All goals should be measurable, be functional, and have an achievement date. Use of the *Guide to Physical Therapist Practice*[1] would be helpful to identify preferred practice patterns and aid in the organization of documentation.

What other information would be helpful for establishing goals and outcomes? And how might the information be obtained?

History information could be obtained by interviewing the patient unless cognition was a problem, in which case the responsible family member could be contacted. Baseline examination data are needed to establish measurable goals.[2]

According to Randall and McEwen,[3] to identify functional goals, it is helpful to understand the patient's activities as well as where they occur, and to establish goals that correspond to the patient's desired outcome. In this case, the documentation does not support the development of functional goals that are specific to the patient's needs.

Further Screening Before Intervention

The most recent physical therapy progress report indicated that the patient complained of headaches, received therapy b.i.d. 5×/week, and improved ambulation with a walker from 20 feet × 2 with standby assistance to 100 to 120 feet with contact guard assistance. Transfers required minimal assistance for sit to stand with verbal cues to move forward in the chair and for walker placement. No goals or contraindications to treatment were described. The therapist indicated that the patient could return home with support if pain decreased.

The physical therapy progress report lacked a clear indication of patient management and what skilled intervention was provided. Nursing interviews revealed concerns regarding nutritional intake and social isolation.

Based on the available information, does the patient demonstrate the potential to return home independently, or is extended care a realistic expectation? How might one proceed with care for this patient and why?

In this case, the therapist recognized a reexamination was warranted as data were lacking and the patient's goals were undefined. Areas previously not addressed in the physical therapy documentation were explored, and the patient, along with his representative, helped formulate the criteria for his return to home. After reexamination, the patient demonstrated a renewed interest in the quality of his performance. He achieved his goals within 3 weeks and returned home with supportive services.

Summary

The relationship between the therapist and patient is important to achieving successful outcomes. Effective documentation will aid the exchange of information and delivery of efficient care. Baker et al[4] found that therapists seek to involve their patients in establishing goals and determining outcomes, but do not maximize the existing potential for this involvement. This finding would seem true in this case study, because the patient's lack of involvement in establishing goals and a limited understanding of the patient's total needs may have delayed the patient's return to home and hindered the transition of care to another therapist.

REFERENCES

1. American Physical Therapy Association: Guide to physical therapist practice, second edition, *Phys Ther* 81:1, 2001.
2. Baeten AM, Moran ML, Phillippi LM: *Documenting physical therapy: the reviewer perspective.* Boston: Butterworth-Heinemann, 1999, p 14.
3. Randall KE, McEwen IR: Writing patient-centered functional goals, *Phys Ther* 80:1199, 2000.
4. Baker SM, Marshak HH, Rice GT, Zimmerman GJ: Patient participation in physical therapy goal setting, *Phys Ther* 81:1126, 2001.

The reader will be able to:

1. Describe how to manage a physical therapy referral with an inappropriate diagnosis.
2. Describe how to utilize a home exercise program with a patient with limited physical therapy visits.
3. Identify the symptoms of coccygodynia.

The reader should know that a 34-year-old woman whose medical diagnosis was low back pain was referred for outpatient physical therapy.

Examination

HISTORY

On interview, the patient reported symptoms including pain in the coccyx area that increased after sitting for a prolonged period and then arising. She also reported pain in the buttocks and sacroiliac joint areas. The symptoms began after she gave birth to twins vaginally 4 months earlier. She initially sought medical treatment 2 months after the birth. Medical intervention at that point included radiographs of the pelvis that were unremarkable, a prescription for Vioxx to relieve pain, and a donut pillow for sitting. She continued to experience symptoms of pain, which made it difficult to sit to feed her twins.

Systems Review

Vital signs were normal.

Tests and Measures

Observation revealed that the patient had a sitting posture of rounded shoulders, forward head tilt, and posterior pelvic tilt with most weight-bearing on the coccyx. Palpation revealed trigger points over the area of the piriformis, gluteus maximus, and levator ani. Intravaginal palpation revealed increased resting tone of the levator ani and 5/5

strength of the muscles of pelvic floor.[1] Manual muscle testing of the hip complex was normal.

Evaluation

At the time of referral, a physician had diagnosed the patient with low back pain and recommended moist heat and ultrasound therapy to the lumbar and sacral spine and lumbar stabilization exercises. On physical therapy examination, signs and symptoms were consistent with coccygodynia (painful coccyx), which in this case resulted from injury to the coccyx area from the passage of the fetuses through the birth canal. Based on these findings, treatment of the lumbar spine was not an appropriate intervention.[2] The physical therapy diagnosis was established as muscle spasm.

Diagnosis

Practice Pattern 4D: Impaired Joint Mobility, Motor Function, Muscle Performance, and Range of Motion Associated With Connective Tissue Dysfunction.[3]

How should a physical therapist proceed? What are appropriate interventions?

Prognosis (Including Plan of Care)

The therapist recommended that the patient be seen three times a week for 4 weeks. The plan of care included soft tissue mobilization to the buttocks and area of piriformis and friction massage to trigger points in the levator ani. Biofeedback was incorporated into the plan to work on decreasing the resting tone of the levator ani utilizing a rectal electrode. In addition, postural training was included to encourage the patient to sit with her weight on the ischial tuberosities rather than the coccyx. The therapist recommended that the patient discontinue using the donut pillow and instead use a coccyx cutout wedge cushion when sitting for a prolonged period, such as when feeding her babies.

Intervention

COORDINATION, COMMUNICATION, AND DOCUMENTATION

Unfortunately, the demand of being a mother to 4-month-old twins limited the patient's ability to attend therapy three times a week. The therapist and patient opted for a treatment program of once-weekly visits complemented by a home program. The patient felt that this was practical and agreed to perform the home program two to three times a week.

The physical therapist also recognized the need to communicate findings to the patient's physician. The therapist contacted the physician via telephone and letter and detailed the findings from the physical therapy examination.

PATIENT/CLIENT-RELATED INSTRUCTION

The therapist recommended a home exercise program of self- or partner massage to the piriformis, stretching of the piriformis, and friction massage of trigger points in the levator ani (see Figure 2-1). This was to be followed by a session of biofeedback for the levator ani utilizing a portable biofeedback machine with an anal electrode.

Outcome

The patient and her husband attended a treatment session together for instruction in self- and partner massage, as well as home use of

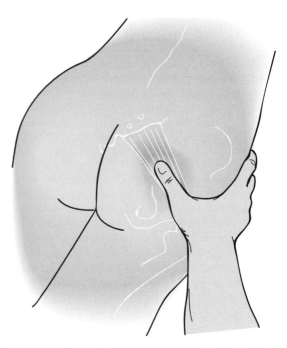

FIGURE 2-1 Partner massage of the piriformis muscle.

the portable biofeedback machine. The patient adhered to the home exercise program two times a week and consistently attended physical therapy treatment sessions for 4 weeks. Symptoms of pain resolved, and the patient was able to feed her twins with a 5-minute break in between children. The posture of rounded shoulders and forward head persisted, so the therapist discharged the patient with a modified home exercise program to include thoracic and cervical posture exercises and recommendations for patient and child positioning during feeding to decrease back strain.

Discussion

Coccygodynia, or coccydynia, is a disorder commonly classified under the diagnosis of pelvic pain, but it may be mistakenly diagnosed as low back pain or sacroiliac joint pain, because pain may refer to the sacroiliac or lumbar areas.[4] Because coccygodynia refers to a specific symptom (pain), it can have different causes. It commonly results from a fall onto the buttocks or trauma during childbirth, causing a partial dislocation of a joint in the coccyx or overstretching of the ligaments and muscles attached to the coccyx.[2,5] Muscle spasm and pain in the tissues around the coccyx may result. The symptom of pain increases when sitting for a prolonged period or when making bed or chair transfers. Therefore, it is important to address the soft tissue injury and resultant impairments in a case such as this.

Injury to the muscles, ligaments, and connective tissue of the pelvis is common during vaginal deliveries as well as during the months leading up to the delivery. Increased ligament laxity, posture alterations, and increased demand on the pelvic floor to support the viscera may lead to musculoskeletal damage. The changes occurring during pregnancy and delivery must be considered when examining and evaluating patients in the antenatal and postnatal period.

Massage, biofeedback, and postural training were the treatments of choice for this patient to decrease muscle spasm in the piriformis, levator ani, and gluteus maximus. The donut pillow may have been exacerbating the patient's symptoms by distributing weight onto the coccyx and promoting a posterior pelvic tilt while sitting. A wedge-shaped cushion with a coccyx cutout would be much more appropriate for this patient, because it takes weight off of the coccyx and redistributes weight to the thighs while encouraging a more appropriate position of the pelvis.

Stretching became part of the patient's home exercise program to relieve some of the pain and spasm in the piriformis. The piriformis may shorten and develop spasms during pregnancy because of the altered position of the lower extremity and an altered gait pattern. In this case it was contributing to the patient's pelvic pain and general increase in tone of the pelvic floor muscles.

REFERENCES

1. Wilder E (ed): *The gynecological manual*, Alexandria, VA: American Physical Therapy Association, 1997.
2. Sapsford R, Bullock-Saxton J, Markwell S (eds): *Women's health: a textbook for physiotherapists*, London: WB Saunders, 1998.
3. American Physical Therapy Association: Guide to physical therapist practice, second edition, *Phys Ther* 81:1, 2001.
4. Stephenson RG, O'Connor LJ: *Obstetric and gynecologic care in physical therapy* (ed 2), Thorofare, NJ: Slack, 2000.
5. Hall CM, Brody LT: *Therapeutic exercise: moving toward function*, Philadelphia: Lippincott Williams & Wilkins, 1999.

Case 3

LEARNING OBJECTIVES

The reader will be able to:

1. Identify the roles of the academician, clinician, and student in dealing with difficult issues in clinical education.

2. Develop a rationale for facilitating active student participation in the design of a remediation plan for clinical education.

The reader should know that a 22-year-old student in the final year of an entry-level 5-year Master of Science in Physical Therapy program was asked to leave the fourth affiliation 4 weeks into a 6-week experience due to patient safety concerns. Visual analog scale markings and clinical instructor comments scored the student below established grading criteria for this level affiliation on the Clinical Performance Instrument (CPI).[1] Primary areas of deficiency were safety, professional behavior, professional demeanor, and communication criteria. The student actively worked with the academic Director of Clinical Education (DCE) to design and participate in a remedial plan. After completing the scheduled remediation activities, the student returned to clinical education and successfully completed the remaining two 6-week affiliations with entry-level scores on the visual analog scale and positive comments from the clinical instructors on safety, professionalism, and communication criteria.

This case is discussed within the framework of the Guide to Physical Therapist Practice[2] elements of patient/client management. The student's ability to function as a competent physical therapy practitioner is the desired outcome. The elements of the model are applied as follows: The student's clinical performance on affiliation is "examined," competence is "evaluated," causes of deficient performance are "diagnosed," the student's optimal level of function and the time needed to achieve that level are "prognosed," activities to promote improved performance are designed (intervention), clinical performance is "reexamined," and "outcomes" are discussed.

Did the student have any issues on previous affiliations? What were the concerns that led to removal?

This student had demonstrated acceptable academic and laboratory performance on examination in individual courses in the program. Faculty evaluation determined acceptable readiness[3] for clinical education based on completed coursework. The clinical instructors evaluated clinical performance and identified problems in the student's development of appropriate professional communication skills and demeanor on the second and third clinical affiliations. After each of these affiliations, the faculty diagnosed the student's needs and designed and directed interventions in the form of remedial plans that the student completed. Despite remediation, similar concerns were raised with reexamination of performance on subsequent clinical education experiences.

During the fourth clinical education affiliation, the faculty planned an early site visit to examine the student's performance. Issues identified by the Clinical Instructor (CI) and Center Coordinator of Clinical Education (CCCE) during the visit were consistent with previously identified issues of communication and professionalism. Studies[4,5] have revealed that behavior in these areas can be indicative of success or failure in clinical education. The academic and clinical faculty discussed the need for change with the student and emphasized the importance of these skills in providing effective patient care. After the faculty visit, the student's performance deteriorated. A learning contract was implemented with CI, CCCE, and DCE input to clarify the level of performance that the student needed to achieve. As examined by the clinical faculty, the student's performance continued to deteriorate. Five documented safety incidents occurred in a 2-day period. These incidents included failure to ascertain a weight-bearing status and proceeding with intervention without first reviewing medical imaging reports.

The site evaluated the situation and asked that the student be removed from the affiliation. The student expressed an inability to perform and an awareness that skills were not improving. The academic program concurred with the site that, given the identified problems, this student was not safe and needed to be removed.

Given the above-described situation, the student could choose to attempt another affiliation immediately, to remediate pertinent issues and then participate in another affil-iation, or to take some time off and resume study next year. Which of these alternatives was chosen? Why?

The clinical instructor provided the academic program with a "final" CPI report and copies of the safety incident reports (evaluation). These reports contained specific examples of performance areas that were not acceptable. The student went home and was asked to take some time to reflect on clinical performance, examine specific situations, and evaluate reasons for the poor performance. Based on established grading criteria, the CPI's comments, and input from the CI and CCCE, the DCE evaluated the data and assigned a "fail" grade for this pass/fail course. Options were discussed, and the student expressed a clear desire to become a competent physical therapist and apply effort to remediate the pertinent issues in a timely manner.

The DCE's evaluation of the data revealed that similar issues were increasing in intensity despite faculty-directed attempts to improve the student's performance. It was decided that the student needed to take

responsibility for performance and identify how to improve it. This could be equated to the diagnosis and prognosis elements of the patient/client management model in the *Guide to Physical Therapist Practice.*[2] The student was asked to diagnose the cause of deficient performance and prognose the ability to be a competent physical therapist. The DCE's role involved facilitation and coordination. With time and coaching to express individual needs, the student was able to identify areas to remediate. The DCE and the student worked together to design a written plan to address needs (plan of care) with specific activities (interventions) that included a time frame for completion (prognosis). The DCE monitored the student's progress (reexamination) toward fulfilling these activities. Together, the DCE and the student agreed that successful completion of the interventions would indicate a readiness to participate in another affiliation.

What specific interventions could be included to address the areas of deficient clinical performance?

The student was able to articulate an inability to adopt professional behaviors and use them in the clinic (evaluation). After reflecting on performance, the student realized a desire to "be everyone's friend" and "do what the CI wanted." The student became aware of personal actions that were an attempt to mold behavior to fit what was learned in school and what was perceived as being desired by the clinic. However, there was a lack of depth and a lack of what the student termed the necessary "thought processes" for the student to become a competent physical therapist (diagnosis). The student expressed a desire to succeed and a motivation to modify performance (prognosis). When asked to identify ways in which growth might occur in this area, the student outlined a remediation plan (intervention) that included the following actions:

1. Perform clinical observation of a practicing physical therapist. The student felt that volunteering in a physical therapy clinic

would allow observation of professionalism, communication, and documentation without the pressure to perform. This would help the student identify specific behaviors that professionalism entails. The student felt that 4 weeks of observation could provide the knowledge needed to develop appropriate "thought processes" (a term that the student used repeatedly when describing the evaluation of performance deficits).

2. Read a textbook on professional communications. Based on knowledge of available resources that matched the student's needs, the DCE proposed suggested readings to the student. After reviewing several options, *Health Professional and Patient Interaction*[6] was selected. The student was to read this text and incorporate the knowledge gained into the development of personal thought processes needed to be a physical therapist.

3. Perform self-assessment and implement the knowledge gained. The student and DCE agreed that there were lessons to be learned from the failed affiliation. The student needed to identify behaviors that had caused problems, articulate what could have prevented issues from occurring and discuss how to behave more competently. The student would define in writing[7] the "thought processes" that were needed, identify and group criteria from the CPI and the objectives for clinical education under each process, and write clinical actions that would enhance effectiveness. Student reflection on personal professional development[8] combined with this activity led the student to outline concrete steps that would be used to advance professionalism.

4. Provide practical application of the knowledge gained. The student expressed a desire to practice new skills before returning to a formal clinical education experience. Working together, the student and DCE decided that paper cases and a practical skill check would be valuable. Paper cases were designed to give the student practice in designing appropriate interventions, setting realistic goals, and documenting hypothetical treatment sessions. The student also agreed to complete a "checkout" of mobility skills with a faculty member, demonstrating skill competency and safety in transfers, bed mobility, and gait training. Modification of interventions and discussion of rationales for treatment based on changing patient scenarios would be included.

5. Set clear, measurable objectives for the next clinical experience. The student set goals for the volunteer observation and for the repeat clinical education experience.

What are potential outcomes demonstrating student competency?

The student completed the remedial plan within the established time frame. The DCE examined the student's content for accuracy and development (reexamination) and determined the student's apparent readiness to return to the clinic. A repeat affiliation was scheduled at a site that (as requested by the student) was fully aware of the student's specific needs. The CI examined the student's performance and evaluated his competency during the affiliation. At midterm and final CPI assessments, the CI discerned appropriate safety, professionalism, and communication performance. The DCE reexamined this performance in the context of previously identified issues and awarded a grade of "pass" for the affiliation. The student then progressed to the fifth and final affiliation with full disclosure to the CI as to the competency areas being emphasized. The student actively sought feedback from the clinician in specific situations and diligently modified his performance to improve competency. At completion of the final affiliation, the student earned positive comments and entry-level performance on all criteria of the CPI. The student went on to successfully pass the state licensing boards and secure full-time employment as a physical therapist. In a follow-up interview, the student concluded that taking responsibility for identifying needs and designing the remediation activities were effective in altering performance as a clinician and achieving competency.

REFERENCES

1. American Physical Therapy Association: *Physical therapy clinical performance instruments.* Alexandria, VA: American Physical Therapy Association, 1998.
2. American Physical Therapy Association: Guide to physical therapist practice, second edition, *Phys Ther* 81:1, 2001.
3. Watson CJ, Barnes CA, Williamson JW: Determinants of clinical performance in a physical therapy program, *J Allied Health* 29:150, 2000.
4. Hayes K, Huber G, Rogers J, Sanders B: Behaviors that cause clinical instructors to question the clinical competence of physical therapist students, *Phys Ther* 79:653, 1999.
5. Gutman SA, McCreedy P, Heisler P: Student level II fieldwork failure: strategies for intervention, *Am J Occup Ther* 52:143, 1998.
6. Purtilo R, Haddad A: *Health professional and patient interaction* (ed 5), Philadelphia, PA: WB Saunders, 1996.
7. Hobson E: Encouraging self-assessment writing as active learning. In Sutherland TE, Bonwell CC (eds): *Using active learning in college classes: a range of options for faculty*, San Francisco: Jossey-Bass, 1996, 45.
8. May WW, Morgan BJ, Lemke JC, Karst GM, Stone HL: Model for ability-based assessment in physical therapy education, *J Phys Ther Ed* 9:3, 1995.

LEARNING OBJECTIVES

The reader will be able to:

1. Identify characteristics in this case that made an intense home exercise program appropriate.

2. Discuss the benefits of providing therapy in the home environment.

The reader should know that an outpatient physical therapist was seeing a 14-year-old female diagnosed with spastic cerebral palsy (CP). The patient was being seen once a month for 30 minutes. The outpatient physical therapist was frustrated with a lack of improvement/progress in the patient's ambulation. The patient was also being treated by a physical therapist at her school, who was seeing her once a week for 30 minutes. Communication between the two therapists suggested that the patient's progress in all areas of functioning had plateaued over the last year. The patient, a high school freshman, would like to attend her first high school social (a dance) in approximately 4 weeks. The patient requested that the therapist assist her with improving her walking so that she could walk into her first social at school. The patient and her mother also voiced a goal to increase the patient's ability to ambulate safely within her house.

Examination

HISTORY

The patient was the sole survivor of a twin pregnancy, delivered secondary to fetal distress at 28 weeks' gestation via cesarean section. She spent 4 months in the neonatal intensive care unit, with history of ventilation, bronchial pulmonary dysplasia, intercranial bleeding (grade IV), and severe feeding problems. The patient was diagnosed with spastic diplegic CP with left hemiplegia by age 3 years. She underwent a dorsal rhizotomy at age 6 and right hip reconstruction at age 13. Before the right hip reconstruction surgery, the patient was a community ambulator with one forearm crutch; after the surgery, she used a power chair for mobility in the community and at school. The patient also had a history of asthma and seizures, which were controlled with Albuterol p.r.n. and Tegretol.

The patient lives in a single-parent family with three younger siblings. The patient's mother is employed and works the second shift, and so is unavailable after school to assist the patient. In addition, the three younger siblings interfere with the patient's ambulation at home and constitute a potential safety hazard for ambulation.

What baseline data were necessary?

SYSTEMS REVIEW/TESTS AND MEASURES

The patient was initially ambulating with large base quad cane for 10 feet on carpeted surfaces with minimum to moderate assistance. She was ambulating exclusively into/out of the bathroom and with therapy at school (once per week). She used a power wheelchair for the remainder of the day for mobility.

Cardiovascular system. Initially, the patient demonstrated a high oxygen saturation level (95% to 97%) before, during, and 1 minute after ambulating 10 feet. Immediately after ambulation, the patient demonstrated an increased breathing rate and breathing effort, with a recovery time of 2 to 3 minutes. Her heart rate increased from 89 beats per minute (bpm) before walking to 167 bpm immediately after ambulating 10 feet.

Musculoskeletal system. The patient wore bilateral single-axis molded ankle foot orthoses (AFOs) for medial/lateral instability at her ankle. Range-of-motion (ROM) measurements were assessed with a goniometer.

TABLE 4-1
GONIOMETRIC RANGE OF MOTION MEASURES

RANGE OF MOTION	PREINTERVENTION		POSTINTERVENTION	
	LEFT	RIGHT	LEFT	RIGHT
Hip flexion	19° to 131°	24° to 133°	18° to 138°	28° to 142°
Hip extension	–19°	–24°	–18°	–24°
Hip abduction	0° to 35°	0° to 17°	0° to 38°	0° to 16°
Hip adduction	0° to 10°	0° to 7°	0° to 10°	0° to 8°
Knee flexion	26° to 110°	17° to 112°	19° to 121°	12° to 131°
Knee extension	–26°	–17°	–19°	–12°
Ankle dorsiflexion	0° to 3°	0° to 1°	0° to 6°	0° to 5°
Ankle plantarflexion	0° to 46°	0° to 49°	0° to 46°	0° to 50°

Generally, ROM measurements were limited throughout both lower extremities, especially at the ends of ROM in most directions. However, ROM was not felt to be limiting function. Specific pretest ROM data are given in Table 4-1. Muscle strength was assessed with a dynamometer (Nicholas Manual Muscle Tester; Lafayette Instrument Company, North Lafayette, Indiana); pretest values are listed in Table 4-2. Strength was measured three times, and these measures were averaged. Generally, strength was significantly decreased, with the right lower extremity weaker than the left lower extremity.

Neuromuscular system. A pedograph (footprint analysis) and stop-watch were used to assess velocity of gait, cadence, stride length, right and left step length, and base of support. The stride length, step length, and base of support values reflect the average of three steps taken with each leg. The results of this testing are given in Table 4-3. Generally, cadence and velocity were greatly reduced, with step length shorter in the right lower extremity and a large base of support.

In addition to the pedograph, active infrared markers were placed on the patient's right lower extremity, and a motion analysis system (CODA[mpx30]; Charnwood Dynamics Limited, Leicestershire, U.K.) was used to determine joint angles in the right lower extremity during gait. Initially, the patient demonstrated a maximum hip extension of –23 degrees and maximum hip flexion of 33 degrees, a maximum knee valgus flexion of 75 degrees, and a maximum ankle flexion of 62 degrees of eversion and 43 degrees of inversion.

The BERG Balance Scale[1] was used to evaluate initial functional balance skill. The patient's BERG score was initially 23/56. The patient did well with sitting items, had problems with standing items, and was unable to perform single-leg stance activities.

Behavioral assessment. The Activity-Specific Balance Confidence (ABC) Scale[2] was modified to fit the patient and used to measure her confidence in her ability to function in her environment. Results of the initial ABC are reported in Table 4-4.

What were the primary factors limiting the patient's ambulation?

Evaluation

After the examination and discussion with the patient and her mother, the therapist determined that the major limitations to returning to household and limited community ambulation were:

1. Decreased endurance
2. Decreased strength
3. Lack of opportunity to safely practice
4. Decreased confidence
5. Lack of a home exercise/ambulation program.

TABLE 4-2
DYNAMOMETER MEASURES IN *N*

STRENGTH (*N*)	PREINTERVENTION		IMMEDIATELY POSTINTERVENTION		2 WEEKS POSTINTERVENTION		4 WEEKS POSTINTERVENTION	
	LEFT	RIGHT	LEFT	RIGHT	LEFT	RIGHT	LEFT	RIGHT
Hip flexion	4.01	1.89	3.41	2.02	6.60	3.73	8.97	6.37
Hip extension	1.41	.53	1.11	.37	2.70	2.13	4.97	3.00
Hip abduction	1.74	.50	2.23	1.79	4.47	3.87	5.80	5.20
Hip adduction	3.94	3.86	5.59	4.68	10.00	9.80	9.90	8.23
Knee extension	1.23	2.52	2.41	2.58	4.43	4.10	4.37	6.20

TABLE 4-3
PEDOGRAPH DATA

PEDOGRAPH DATA	VELOCITY (M/MIN)	CADENCE (STEPS/MIN)	STRIDE LENGTH (CM)	STEP LENGTH (CM)		BASE OF SUPPORT (CM)
				LEFT	RIGHT	
Preintervention	15.47	21.46	61.47	41.63	20.42	20.02
Immediately postintervention	25.83	22.95	76.78	56.03	21.34	24.23
2 weeks postintervention	22.09	26.46	72.24	44.60	27.15	23.19
4 weeks postintervention	26.78	25.66	73.56	52.76	28.23	23.02
Normal range	Variable	90–120	70–82	35–41	35–41	5–10

Diagnosis

Practice Pattern 5C: Impaired Motor Function and Sensory Integrity Associated with Nonprogressive Disorders of the Central Nervous System—Congenital Origin or Acquired in Infancy or Childhood.[6]

Prognosis (including plan of care)

After the examination, the therapist concluded that this 14-year-old girl was capable of increasing her ability to ambulate in her home and at school and to ambulate into her first high school social in 4 weeks secondary to high motivation and availability of an intense home therapy program over the next 4 weeks.

What research-based evidence could be used to develop a plan of care?

Based on research by Bower et al,[3] the therapist planned a short period of intense intervention to promote functional gains in this patient. She was seen in her home five times during week 1, three times during week 2, two times during week 3, and one time during week 4. The patient was contacted daily, either with a home visit or via telephone. A home exercise program was developed to improve the functional and impairment-level problems associated with ambulation. The patient was given an easy-to-read chart with check-off boxes for each part of the exercise program to help her keep a written record of her progress for the month-long intense intervention program. Additional check-off charts were provided each month after the intense intervention phase.

TABLE 4-4
RESULTS OF ABC ASSESSMENT BOTH PRE AND POSTINTERVENTION

How confident are you that you will not lose your balance or become unsteady when you …	Pretest	Posttest
Walk around the house?	25%	60%
Bend over and pick up an object from the floor?	0%	0%
Reach for a video off a shelf at eye level?	0%	25%
Walk from the front door of your house to a car parked in the driveway?	35%	40%
Get into or out of a car?	60%	75%
Walk in a crowded place where people may bump into you?	0%	10%
Walk outside on the grass or in your yard?	0%	80%

Intervention

The patient was seen in her home for a program of walking inside and outside of the house. The home program included pedaling on a foot bike; work on weight shifting in standing and functional reaching; stretching of hamstrings, hip flexors, and knee extensors; and strengthening exercises for hip flexion, abduction, and adduction and knee extension. The home program was designed to take 15 to 20 minutes each day, based on the work of Schreiber et al.[4] In this intervention, involvement of family members was limited due to the mother's work schedule and the siblings' young age. Reassessment was planned for immediately after completion of the intense intervention phase, and then 2 weeks and 4 weeks postintervention.

Reexamination

CARDIOVASCULAR SYSTEM

The patient's oxygen saturation levels continued to remain above 95% throughout periods of ambulation. Immediately after ambulation, the patient demonstrated no increased breathing rate or increased breathing effort, and no recovery time was needed. Heart rate was now 82 to 86 bpm before ambulating and 91 to 100 bpm after ambulating for 50 feet. These cardiovascular improvements, seen immediately postintervention, were maintained the 2-week and 4-week postintervention reassessments.

MUSCULOSKELETAL SYSTEM

No significant changes in ROM were noted immediately postintervention (see Table 4-1). No changes in ROM were expected, because the original ROM was sufficient to allow the patient to ambulate and this was not a major focus of the home exercise program. ROM was not remeasured at the 2-week and 4-week postintervention follow-ups.

Strength measurement demonstrated an improvement immediately postintervention; however, these improvements continued and even increased over the subsequent 4 weeks. Changes in strength were found in all muscles assessed 4 weeks postintervention.

NEUROMUSCULAR SYSTEM

Pedograph data demonstrated an increase in ambulation velocity, cadence, stride length, and step length (see Table 4-3). A small increase in base of support was also demonstrated, but this was thought to be the result of improved symmetry in the lower extremity (i.e., decreased valgus in the right lower extremity). (Normal values are based on those listed in Magee's *Orthopedic Physical Assessment.*[5])

Changes in gait were also observed in the joints of the right lower extremity during ambulation. Based on the CODA movement analysis system, the hip maximum range increased to 42 degrees of flexion and −18 degrees of extension, maximum knee valgus decreased to 45 degrees, and maximum ankle motion decreased to 54 degrees of eversion and 1 degree of inversion.

The patient's Berg balance scale score also increased, to 33/56 immediately postintervention and then to 35/56 at 4 weeks postintervention. Specifically, improvements were observed in the following areas: standing unsupported, performing transfers, standing with feet together, reaching forward with outstretched arms, retrieving an object from the floor, turning to look behind, and turning 360 degrees.

By the end of the first week of intervention in the home, the patient was independent in performing her home exercise program except for needing minimum assistance to secure her feet on the foot bike. In the second week, during one of the home visits, the patient reported that "I am walking so much straighter and feel so much better when I walk."

BEHAVIORAL ASSESSMENT

Reassessment with the modified version of the ABC scale demonstrated the patient's increase in confidence in such activities as walking around the house, reaching for her videos off her shelf in her room, walking from her front door to a car in the driveway, getting into or out of a car, walking in a crowded place where she could be bumped, and walking outside in her own yard (see Table 4-4). The ABC test was not readministered at the 2-week or 4-week postintervention assessment.

Outcome

The patient improved her ability to ambulate in her home and at school (although limited by staff availability to assist and supervise), and was able to ambulate into her first high school social. The patient and her peers and family were able to share in her success in ambulating 90 feet with a quad cane and standby assistance into the dance. The social support experienced by the patient at this school event made a significant impact on her confidence. She stated numerous times how much stronger she felt and how excited she was about the improvements that she had made. The patient was given charts to continue her home exercise program, and her outpatient therapist continued to follow her program and update it as needed.

Discussion

A home exercise program as an adjunct to physical therapy intervention is important to optimize functional gains within the natural environment. To be effective, an exercise program must be easy to follow and become part of the daily routine. Ideally, successful programs should involve family members to help motivate and guide the child. In this case, parental involvement was limited by the mother's employment status, and it was not appropriate to seek sibling assistance. A limited intense period of physical therapy allowed this patient to become independent in her home exercise program, gave her an ability to function in her natural environment, and positively impacted her social interaction with her peers.

REFERENCES

1. Berg KO, Wood-Dauphinee SL, Williams JI, et al: Measuring balance in the elderly: preliminary development of an instrument, *Physiother Can* 41:304, 1998.
2. Powell LE, Myers AM: The activities-specific balance confidence (ABC) scale, *J Gerontol A Biol Sci Med Sci* 50:28, 1995.
3. Bower E, McLennan DL, Arney J, Campbell MJ: A randomized controlled trial of different intensities of physiotherapy and different goal-setting procedures in 44 children with cerebral palsy, *Dev Med Child Neurol* 50:28, 1996.
4. Schreiber JM, Effgen SK, Palisano RJ: Effectiveness of parental collaboration on compliance with a home program, *Pediatr Phys Ther* 7:59, 1995.
5. Magee DJ: *Orthopedic physical assessment*, Philadelphia: WB Saunders, 1997.
6. American Physical Therapy Association: Guide to physical therapist practice, second edition, *Phys Ther* 81:1, 2001.

LEARNING OBJECTIVES

The reader will be able to:

1. Identify the clinical tests necessary to distinguish the various upper extremity symptoms that a patient with cervical radiculopathy may experience.

2. Describe the proper position for the body and equipment during regular office computer use.

3. Discuss the incidence, prognosis, and typical rehabilitation of a patient with cervical radiculopathy.

Examination

HISTORY

The patient was a 47-year-old single white female accountant with a chief complaint of right upper extremity symptoms of 4 months' duration. Her symptoms began insidiously as a tingling and occasionally burning sensation over the lateral forearm, hands, and thumbs. She also complained of a tingling in the right palm, which began 2 months earlier. She reported that she began dropping things 2 weeks earlier, and this caused her to seek medical attention.

The forearm and thumb symptoms were worse at the end of the day, after prolonged sitting or computer use, or after looking up for more than 5 minutes. The tingling in the palms awakened her after 1 hour of sleep and commonly occurred after 30 minutes of computer use.

The patient's past medical history included a right radial head fracture at age 21 and a rear-end auto collision at age 35. She had no ongoing complaints from either of those episodes before the onset of the current symptoms. She reported jogging 3 miles per day. Cervical radiographs showed moderate degenerative changes at C5-6 bilaterally and mild changes at C4-5 and C6-7. Magnetic resonance imaging showed osteophyte formation in the region of the right C5-6 neural foramen, and an electromyelography study showed mild sensory loss in the right median nerve distribution and the lateral forearm.

Weakness was also noted in the thenar muscles.

SYSTEMS REVIEW

Integumentary system. The patient exhibited decreased sensation to pinprick at the tip of the right thumb. She did not complain of any recent bruising or contact discoloration from the time that symptoms developed.

Musculoskeletal system

Gross sym-metry. The patient presented with a marked forward head posture and a prominent angle at the cervical-thoracic (CT) junction. The upper extremities were internally rotated, with visible tightness of the anterior cervical and both upper trapezius muscles. There was poor muscle definition of the posterior scapular muscles and slight atrophy of the right thenar muscles.

Palpation. Palpation of the cervical spine at C5-7 on the right elicited tenderness and a reproduction of right forearm symptoms. Accessory movements of the cervical spine revealed hypomobility at C1-2, especially during right rotation. Spinal segments at C3-5 were assessed as hypermobile, those at C6-7 could not be assessed because of irritability of the segment, and those at C7-T3 were found to be hypomobile.

There was increased muscle tightness of the right cervical paravertebral muscles and parascapular muscles, especially the sternocleidomastoid, levator scapulae, and scalenes. There was generalized tightness bilaterally in the flexor muscles of forearms, identified by a "ropelike" feeling.

Joint range of motion. Cervical flexion was limited by 50% with no reversal of cervical lordosis. Cervical extension was full, but no motion occurred below the CT junction. There was an increase in right forearm symptoms with prolonged cervical extension. Side flexion to the right was 75% full range without an increase in symptoms and side flexion to the left was 50% of full range but eased the symptoms. Cervical rotation to the right was only 40% of full range, limited by increased symptoms in the right forearm. Cervical rotation to the left was 80% of normal range, and the symptoms in the right forearm decreased.

Range of motion of the shoulders and the left elbow was within normal limits. Flexion of the right elbow was full, extension was –7 degrees, and pronation and supination were both 80 degrees. Bilateral extension of the wrists was measured at 60 degrees with the fingers flexed and 45 degrees with the fingers extended.

Strength. Weakness was noted in the abductor (3/5) and extensor (4/5) pollicis brevis muscles of the right thumb. No other weakness was observed bilaterally. Cervical motion was limited by the onset of pain and other symptoms, but strength within the available range was within normal limits.

Neurologic system. There was a diminished brachioradialis reflex on the right side compared with the left side. Nerve tension testing utilizing full tension on the median nerve pathway reproduced all symptoms.

Special tests. The Adson's, military, and hyperabduction tests were negative. Phalen's test and Tinel's sign were noted as positive.

From the foregoing information, how were the severity, irritability and nature of the symptoms rated?

The patient's symptoms were considered of moderate severity. The irritability was moderate because of radicular symptoms (in particular, the cervical symptoms), which should almost always be considered irritable until proved otherwise. The nature was identified as C6 cervical radiculopathy with potential secondary carpal tunnel syndrome, caused by the restricted mobility of the right elbow and cervical spine secondary to earlier injuries.

Diagnosis

Physical Therapist Practice Pattern 5H: Impaired Motor Function, Peripheral Nerve Integrity, and Sensory Integrity Associated With Nonprogressive Disorders of the Spinal Cord.

Prognosis (including plan of care)

The prognosis for conservative care of the cervical radiculopathy in this patient was considered fair to good, because of motor changes. The prognosis for surgical laminectomy/fusion was considered good; however, surgery would not be considered until conservative management had been attempted. The prognosis for conservative management of the carpal tunnel syndrome was considered good as long as contributing factors were eliminated or managed and if symptoms were caught early. The prognosis for surgical release of the carpal tunnel was considered good.

SHORT-TERM GOALS
The patient will:
1. Have less pain and tenderness arising from the neck by the end of the second week of treatment.
2. Have decreased tingling sensation in the forearm and hand by the end of the first week of treatment.
3. Increase the available range of motion in the cervical region by the end of the fourth week of treatment.
4. Increase strength in the right upper extremity gradually over the course of the treatment sessions.

LONG-TERM GOALS

The patient will:

1. Regain full range of motion in the cervical region by the end of the eighth week of treatment.
2. Have no lasting altered sensation in the right upper extremity 3 months after treatment has concluded.
3. Regain full strength in the right upper extremity by the end of the eighth week of treatment.
4. Develop the knowledge during the first 2 weeks of treatment that will ensure that she avoids situations that will lead to similar symptoms in the future.

Intervention

The patient was given a prescription for a nonsteroidal antiinflammatory drug and referred to physical therapy by her primary care physician. The physician discussed surgical intervention with the patient, consisting of a decompression laminectomy or a spinal fusion. Initial treatment of the cervical radiculopathy began with extensive patient education in sitting posture, computer use with consideration of both cervical position and hand position, sleeping posture, pillow selection, avoidance of static positions, and avoidance of the closed-pack position of the right cervical region. The necessity of attaining and maintaining correct posture during work and activities of daily living was reinforced throughout the treatment sessions.

Cervical traction was used on the first day of treatment, with a very gentle 5 lb of traction applied. Other techniques used to reduce nerve root irritation included Maitland grade I central vertebral pressure techniques directed in a posteroanterior direction. These techniques were applied in 30-second bouts separated by 1-minute rest and reevaluation periods. A total of four bouts were applied. The patient was sent home with a home exercise program that included the open-pack position for symptomatic relief, modified dorsal glides (McKenzie chin retraction exercises) with progression to improved mobility as tolerated, stretching to correct upper quadrant (including the upper extremities) alignment, and frequent stretching breaks during the workday. Exercises for the forearm included gentle extrinsic flexor muscle-strengthening activities accompanied by frequent stretching breaks.

The patient was also given soft tissue mobilization to the right upper quadrant muscles, especially the scalenes, pectoralis minor, sternocleidomastoid, and upper trapezius.

Outcome

The patient stated that the traction initially produced decreased symptoms in the neck followed by decreased symptoms in the forearm. However, she did report increased symptoms immediately after the traction force was removed. The force was decreased for the subsequent sessions such that the patient felt symptomatic relief but did not experience the posttraction exacerbation. The Maitland mobilization techniques produced a reduction in symptoms in the neck and forearm. The patient was very compliant with her home exercise program and took steps at her workplace to rearrange her desk and ensure proper postural alignment.

Reexamination

The patient was treated three times per week for the first 3 weeks and then two times per week for the following 3 weeks. The reexamination was done 6 weeks after the initial examination, at which time the patient's cervical spine mobility had improved, with forward flexion now 70% of normal range but still without reversal of the normal lordosis. Cervical extension was full, with some limited motion at the CT junction. Side flexion to the right was 85% of full range with no increase in symptoms, and side flexion to the left was 60% of full range with a slight decrease in symptoms. Rotation to the right was 60% of normal range with an increase in forearm symptoms, and rotation to the left was 90% of normal range with an associated decrease in symptoms. Accessory motion of the cervical spine was normal for the C1-2 segments, hypermobile for the C3-5 segments, and hypomobile for the C6-7 segments, and C7-T3 had achieved more normalized motion.

Ranges of active elbow flexion and extension were full, and pronation and supination were both 85 degrees actively. Wrist extension was 75 degrees with the fingers flexed and 60 degrees with the fingers extended.

The patient exhibited improved sensation to pinprick at the tip of the right thumb, but weakness (4/5) of the abductor and extensor pollicis brevis muscles persisted. The brachioradialis reflex was approaching normal, and full pressure on the median nerve pathway (plus overpressure) reproduced symptoms in the right forearm. Tinel's sign and Phalen's test remained positive.

How was the patient's knowledge of workplace ergonomics assessed?

Assessment of the patient's knowledge of workplace ergonomics includes the following:
1. The patient was seated at a work station in the clinic.
2. She was asked to state which parts of her posture were not in an optimal position.
3. She then demonstrated how to adjust that work station to specifically suit her body shape and needs.

Discharge Summary

This patient was progressing very well with treatment up to this point and was educated on the need for her to continue with her home exercise program and to continue attending the clinic for at least another 4 to 6 visits. The patient was discharged from the clinic once her maximum pain-free range of motion was achieved at the cervical spine. Symptoms at the forearm and thumb persisted; however, the patient was advised to continue with her exercises and was reviewed every 3 months for the following year.

RECOMMENDED READINGS

Cailliet R: *Neck and arm pain* (ed 2), Philadelphia: FA Davis, 1991.

Maitland G, Hengeveld E, Banks K, English K: *Maitland's vertebral manipulation* (ed 6), Melbourne, Australia: Butterworth Heinemann, 2001.

American Physical Therapy Association: Guide to physical therapist practice, second edition, *Phys Ther* 81:1, 2001.

LEARNING OBJECTIVES

The reader will be able to:

1. Define the term "scoliosis" and identify how the curves that occur in the spinal column are classified.
2. Identify the common postural deviations that occur with idiopathic scoliosis.
3. Discuss the common management principles utilized with patients with idiopathic scoliosis.
4. Identify the role of the physical therapist in the management of idiopathic scoliosis.

Examination

HISTORY

The patient, a 12-year-old white female, was referred to physical therapy by an orthopedic specialist with a diagnosis of idiopathic scoliosis. The referral requested that an exercise program be implemented in conjunction with orthotic management of the spinal curve. The patient's pediatrician initially detected the scoliosis during an annual physical examination. The presenting curve was measured radiographically as a 33-degree right thoracic (T5-11) curve and a 30-degree left lumbar (T11-L4) curve. The patient received a Boston brace 2 weeks before the initial physical therapy examination and was advised to wear the brace 23 hours each day. The patient reported some difficulty getting used to the brace, due to the initial discomfort associated with wearing it and generally feeling self-conscious when wearing it; however, she also reported "no pain" in her back after wearing the brace for 2 weeks.

The patient was in the seventh grade and participated in gym at school but undertook no other extracurricular activities. She was generally healthy, with no previous significant history of musculoskeletal injury. She had not started menses at the time of examination.

SYSTEMS REVIEW

Integumentary system. There was no remarkable findings except for two small slightly reddened areas noted on both iliac crests after the brace was removed. This redness resolved within 10 minutes of doffing the brace.

Musculoskeletal system

Gross symmetry. No leg length discrepancy was seen. Observation from the posterior aspect revealed a thoracic curve with right convexity and a lumbar curve with left convexity. The curvature was generally well compensated for, but the patient presented with her head tilted to the right, her left shoulder lowered, and her left waist fold higher. Her right ribs humped posteriorly on forward bending, and she had a more prominent erector spinae muscle on the right side. Mildly winging scapulae were also apparent bilaterally. Observation from the anterior aspect revealed that the chest wall was more prominent on the left side.

Palpation. No palpable muscle spasm was noted on either side of the spinal column.

Joint range of motion. The lower extremity active range of motion (ROM) was within normal limits with the exception of tight hamstrings, which produced a popliteal angle of 145 degrees bilaterally. Active ROM testing for the trunk identified that forward flexion was decreased by 50% (i.e., the fingertips reaching only the middle of the thighs), lateral flexion to the right was decreased by 30% (i.e., the fingertips just reaching the knee), and rotation to the left was decreased by 30% when compared with the opposite direction.

Strength. In general, the patient's strength was fair to good, with the following measurements noted: gross scores of 4/5 for the upper and lower extremities, 4/5 for the rectus abdominus, and 3/5 for the oblique abdominals, trunk extensors, and scapular muscles.

Other joints. The patient had no complaints at either the hips or knees, with full pain-free ROM available, aside from the specific signs and symptoms previously identified.

Special tests. Both the Thomas test and the Ober test were positive bilaterally, although no objective measure was taken. The patient was independent with dressing and all activities of daily living. She required some assistance to don the brace but was independent with doffing. She was able to walk for 10 minutes on the treadmill at 2.5 mph and level grade. Conversational dyspnea commenced at 7 minutes with a verbal report of fatigue. Values for heart rate and respiratory rate were as given in Table 6-1.

The patient was well compensated, with a right convex thoracic and left convex lumbar curve. Which asymmetries identified were expected for this patient?

The following asymmetries were expected:
- Shoulder lower on the concave side of the thoracic curve.
- Scapula farther away from the spine on the concave side of the thoracic curve.
- Waist folds higher on the concave side of the lumbar curve.
- Iliac crest higher on the concave side of the lumbar curve.
- Rib hump on the convex side of the thoracic curve.

TABLE 6-1
TARGET HEART RATE: 156 TO 169

	RESTING	PEAK	COOL DOWN
Heart rate	78	168	84
Respiratory rate	18	36	24

- More prominent erector spinae musculature on the convex side of the thoracic curve.
- More prominent chest wall on the concave side of the thoracic curve.

Diagnosis

Physical Therapist Practice Patterns 4A: Primary Prevention/Risk Reduction for Skeletal Demineralization, and 4B: Impaired Posture.

Prognosis (including plan of care)

It was anticipated that with time, wearing the brace, and a good home exercise program, the patient would gradually regain a more normal alignment of the spinal column without lasting significant complications. The expected number of visits was between eight and twelve. Initially, the patient was seen for five to six appointments for instruction in the home exercise program, which was designed to improve flexibility and strength as well as to establish an aerobic program. The patient and her parents jointly established a checklist to document compliance with the exercise program and brace use. The patient was followed up every 3 to 4 months to reevaluate and update the exercise program as needed through her growing years.

SHORT-TERM GOALS
The patient will:
1. Become more accustomed to wearing the brace and more accomplished in donning and doffing the brace independently during the first week after the brace is prescribed.
2. Undertake a home exercise program to prevent disuse atrophy associated with brace wear beginning during the second week of treatment and continuing while she attends therapy.
3. Become more physically active while wearing the brace to develop and improve spinal position.

LONG-TERM GOALS

The patient will:

1. Develop increased strength in the trunk muscles and continue to improve her static posture by the end of the eighth week.
2. Increase trunk flexibility, trunk muscle strength, and endurance associated with disuse muscle atrophy by the end of the tenth week.
3. Develop sufficient strength to ensure that improvements in static posture are maintained during dynamic activity continuous from the early stages of treatment until the end of the twelfth week.
4. Gradually decrease her reliance on the brace and become more independent, with maintenance of normal spinal curvature beginning by the tenth week and gradually working toward independence without the brace by the fifteenth week.

Intervention

Initial treatment comprised passive movements of the thoracic and lumbar spinal sections to assess the possibility for the scoliosis to resolve and return to a more appropriate spinal alignment. Once the curve was evaluated to be completely reversible, the patient and her parents were educated as to what constitutes a "normal" spinal position. The end point of the treatment program was identified, and a more specific exercise program was devised to assist the patient in achieving her goals. The exercises were designed such that those muscles on the convex aspect of the curves were contracted to encourage flattening of the concavity on the opposite side of the spine while the muscles on the concave aspect of the curvature were stretched to allow the appropriate movement. There were a number of exercises performed independently by the patient and a number of exercises performed by the patient with her parents' assistance. Electrical stimulation was used on the convex side of the curve (at night) to alter the direction of deformity, decrease pressure on the concave side, and allow for more normal vertebral growth.

Outcome

Initially, the patient was relatively noncompliant with both wearing the brace and performing her exercise program. After some discussion, the patient admitted that she felt very self-conscious wearing the brace and had been teased in school when she wore it.

What steps were taken to encourage the patient to continue to wear the brace and perform the exercise program?

The alternative to wearing the brace— surgical intervention—was discussed with both the patient and her parents. They agreed to try using the brace for at least 6 months to avoid the surgical route.

After wearing the brace and performing her exercises for 3 weeks, the patient stated that she had experienced some discomfort when stretching the trunk muscles on the concave aspect of her curve and also similar discomfort when stretching her hamstrings. The therapist reviewed the patient's stretching technique and determined that the patient was performing her stretching exercises correctly, but too vigorously. At this point, all of the strengthening exercises in the patient's program were also reviewed and any problems were corrected.

Reexamination

On reexamination after 6 weeks, the patient complained of some slight discomfort when stretching and occasional discomfort from wearing the brace but little else. In terms of postural dysfunction, her head no longer tilted to the right, her left shoulder remained slightly lower, and her left waist fold was now equal to her right waist fold. The right rib hump, which occurred posteriorly during forward bending, remained. The prominent erector spinae muscles were also still visible on the right side. The reddening of the iliac crests was not present; however, there were signs of old blister scars.

Active ROM remained within normal limits, and the tightness noted in the hamstrings was decreased somewhat, with the popliteal angles measured at 170 degrees bilaterally. The Thomas and Ober tests were still assessed as slightly positive bilaterally. ROM of the trunk had improved with forward flexion from a decrease of 50% to one of 25%; lateral flexion to the right improved from a decrease of 30% to one of 15%; and rotation to the left improved from a decrease of 30% to one of 15%. Strength measures had apparently improved slightly, but not in all areas. The oblique abdominals, trunk extensors and scapular muscles all improved to 4/5, whereas the upper extremities, lower extremities, and rectus abdominus remained at 4/5.

The patient was now independent with dressing and activities of daily living, including independent donning and doffing of the brace. Her endurance increased to 20 minutes on the treadmill at 2.5 mph on a level grade. Conversational dyspnea commenced at 12 minutes with report of fatigue. There were no significant changes in heart rate or respiratory rate.

Discharge Statement

Discharge from physical therapy did not officially take place; however, after 6 weeks of treatment the patient was given a revised home exercise program, and a return appointment was scheduled for 6 months from that date. The patient was advised to adhere to her exercise program and to contact the therapist if anything untoward occurred before her next appointment.

RECOMMENDED READINGS

Calliet R: *Scoliosis: diagnosis and management*, Philadelphia: FA Davis, 1985.

Campbell SK: *Physical therapy for children.* Philadelphia: WB Saunders, 1994.

Tachdjian MO: *Pediatric orthopedics*, vol 3, Philadelphia: WB Saunders, 1990.

American Physical Therapy Association: Guide to physical therapist practice, second edition, *Phys Ther* 81:1, 2001.

LEARNING OBJECTIVES

The reader will be able to:

1. Identify pertinent information to support a physical therapy diagnosis of inefficient/ineffective movement patterns resulting in greater energy demand to perform tasks.
2. Explore approaches to address energy-conserving devices and movement patterns.
3. Discuss aerobic activity benefits for those who have fatigue as an impediment to quality of life.

The reader should know the patient participated in an outpatient education program for people with multiple sclerosis (MS) and their significant others. Each participant was encouraged to bring questions, concerns, and activity goals to the medical team. The team assessed the patient's physical capabilities and interests, then formulated an activity program congruent with the patient's goals and abilities.

According to the Guide for Physical Therapist Practice,[1] the potential functional limitations or disabilities displayed by patients with MS include deconditioning from a cardio-vascular, neuromuscular, or musculoskeletal deficit that could lead to impaired endurance and progressive loss of function. Neuromuscular difficulties resulting from this patient's disorder included difficulty in coordinating movement related to gait on home, work, or community terrains. This impaired motor function and impaired sensory integrity impeded the patient's ability to perform her employment duties as a software technician because her hands were involved, and she complained of decreased fine motor skills interfering with her ability at the keyboard.

Examination

GENERAL DEMOGRAPHICS

The patient, a 5-foot, 5-inch, 55-year-old female software technician who weighed 149 pounds with a body mass index (BMI) of 24.4, had an 11-year diagnosis of MS (although her symptoms began 16 years earlier). She had a Kurtzke expanded disability status scale (EDSS) score (i.e., disability index) of stage 2, meaning that she had minimal disability, with slight weakness or stiffness, minor gait disturbances, or mild motor disturbances. She was married, lived with a supportive husband, and had two grown daughters who lived in a neighboring state.

What home modifications may have helped this patient to conserve her energy and help create a safe environment for her to work and live in?

The patient's house was equipped with an office so that she could perform her work duties at home without having to go outside. She lived in a three-bedroom, two-bathroom, single-level home. On the outside of the house, there were three steps to both the front and back doors. Handrails were installed on both sets of steps. She was able to go up and down the steep basement steps, but did so only when absolutely necessary.

The patient enjoyed generally good health, although she experienced numbness in her hands and fatigue that required rest. She walked around the house without any assistive devices, but used a straight cane or a cane with a folding seat for outings. She was able to manage her household with her husband's help. At times, she had difficulty managing multiple tasks requiring short-term memory. She participated in physical activity about three days per week, including stretching for

15 minutes and cycling for 10 minutes. In the summer months, she also swam for 1 hour three times a week. The only medications that she took were Avonex (an interferon used to slow disease progression),[2] Evista (for osteoporosis prevention),[3] and aspirin for prevention of heart disease and stroke.

What examination procedures could be included for a patient with MS at Kurtzke stage 2?

TESTS AND MEASURES

The patient's EDSS score was 3.5.[4] Testing of her aerobic capacity on a Schwinn Airdyne cycle ergometer yielded the results given in Table 7-1.

Significant weakness was found in right shoulder abduction, external rotation, and elbow flexion (4/5) and in left shoulder flexion and external rotation (4-/5). In the left leg, strength was assessed at 4/5 in straight-knee hip flexion, 4/5 in hip external rotation, 4-/5 in hip extension, and 3/5 in hip extension. In the right leg, strength was 4/5 in bent-knee hip flexion, hip external rotation, and knee flexion. Strength in trunk flexion was 3/5.[6] A hip flexion contracture of 5 degrees on the left was also noted.[7]

The patient was hyperreflexic in both lower extremities and the left upper extremity, but exhibited no clonus or nystagmus. Her vibratory sense and stereognosis were intact bilaterally, although blunted on the left side.

On ambulation, the patient exhibited a forward head, anterior pelvic tilt, and mild ataxia. She was able to walk 25 feet in 6.3 seconds (the average of two trials), and her score on the Tinetti balance assessment was 25/28, indicating a low risk of falls.[8]

What modifications may enable someone with sensory and cognitive loss (problems with multiprocessing with short-term memory) to perform their computer technical support duties at work?

The patient worked as a software consultant from her home office, where she used an exercise ball as a chair during work. She tried to be as active as possible with cooking, cleaning, gardening, and other activities, but she was limited by her energy levels. She learned to pace herself and to sit with proper posture. At work, she kept a detailed diary of conversations with customers. She stated that others in her position might not need to do this, but that it helped her focus on one problem at a time.

Evaluation

The patient presented as a very functional, well-adjusted woman with minimal physical dysfunction, although she stated she felt "wobbly" on her feet and thus used a straight cane for balance and reassurance. Her weight was within a healthy range, and her balance and gait skills were good. She had weakness in her hips and trunk flexors, which may have contributed to her feeling of insecurity while ambulating on level and unlevel surfaces. She had good exercise tolerance, and was in need of education regarding safe levels of aerobic exercise and daily activity.

TABLE 7-1
AEROBIC CAPACITY TESTING

	RESTING	PEAK	COMMENTS
Heart rate	79	142	Resting ECG showed nonspecific ST changes
Blood pressure	144/90	160/92	Test duration: 6 min
			Peak RPE 7 (1-10 Borg scale)[5]

ECG, Electrocardiogram; *RPE*, rate of perceived exertion.

Diagnosis

Physical Therapist Practice Patterns 5A: Primary Prevention/Risk Reduction for Loss of Balance and Falling, and 5E: Impaired Motor Function and Sensory Integrity Associated with Progressive Disorders of the Central Nervous System.

Prognosis

Few factors that could prolong the need for continued intervention were present in this case. The patient had a consistently supportive husband and employer. Her work setting was adjusted to allow continued employment without interruption resulting from her disorder. She had no comorbidities, she maintained adequate nutrition, and her disorder had not progressed markedly over the past 11 years. She enthusiastically embraced the exercise recommendations.

Intervention

COORDINATION, COMMUNICATION, AND DOCUMENTATION

As part of a multidisciplinary approach, the patient was given a binder in which to place lecture notes and exercise recommendations, as well as any questions that arose during the class times, to maintain a record of what she learned and to help her review material after returning home. The exercise prescription was practiced throughout the educational program, and was provided to the patient in both audiotape and written formats on the last day of the program.

Which interventions for decreasing muscle tone are efficacious for patients with MS?

The exercise program included the following activities:

- Flexibility: Daily stretching with emphasis on the lower back and lower extremities.

- Aerobic: Stationary bike, four to five days per week at a rating of perceived exertion of 3 to 4 (on a scale of 1 to 10), moderate to somewhat hard for 6 minutes. Include warm-up and cool down periods. Increase duration by no more than 10% per week, as tolerated, to 20 minutes.
- Balance and coordination: Swiss ball, pool, or counter exercises, two to three days per week.
- Strength: Abdominal and lower extremity strengthening exercises, two to three days per week.

What strategies could be suggested to improve the endurance of a patient complaining of fatigue after walking with a standard cane for 3 minutes at a moderate speed?

The patient's cane height was adjusted and the hand position altered for thumb and wrist safety (Figure 7-1).

Reexamination

The patient was given a home exercise program and ideas of how to integrate the suggested activities into her life. She was supplied with a log sheet to fill in as she continued her activities. She was to return the completed sheet with her subjective comments to have the exercise prescription modified accordingly.

Outcome

The patient was very aware of her activities during the day and stated that she had a hard time stopping before she became overtired. She improved in monitoring her activities (including rest periods and prioritizing tasks) and was learning to pace herself by keeping a diary of her activities and how she felt. As she controlled her life better, she found that she had more energy and focused on participating in activities that she enjoyed and was able to enjoy them even more.

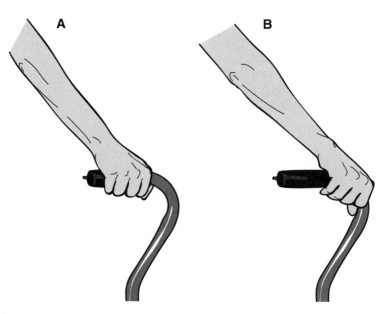

FIGURE 7-1 Hand placement on the cane. **A,** Correct hand placement. **B,** Incorrect hand placement.

REFERENCES

1. American Physical Therapy Association: Guide to physical therapist practice, second edition, *Phys Ther* 81:9, 2001.
2. Rudick RA, Goodkin DE, Jacobs LD, et al: Impact of interferon beta-1a on neurologic disability in relapsing multiple sclerosis, *Neurology* 57(12 Suppl 5):S25, 2001.
3. Barrett-Connor E: Raloxifene: Risks and benefits, *Ann N Y Acad Sci* 949:295, 2001.
4. Kurtzke J: Rating neurological impairment in multiple sclerosis: an expanded disability status scale (EDSS), *Neurology* 33:1444, 1983.
5. Stuifbergen AK: Physical activity and perceived health status in persons with multiple sclerosis, *J Neurosci Nurs* 29:238, 1997.
6. Kendall FP, McCreary EK: *Muscle testing and function* (ed 3), Baltimore: Williams & Wilkins, 1983.
7. Hislop HJ, Montgomery J, Connelly, B: *Daniels and Worthingham's muscle testing: Techniques of manual examination* (ed 6), Philadelphia: WB Saunders, 1995.
8. Berg KO, Maki BE, Williams JI, et al: Clinical and laboratory measures of postural balance in an elderly population, *Arch Phys Med Rehab* 73:1073, 1992.

LEARNING OBJECTIVES

The reader will be able to:

1. Classify a patient with Bell's palsy according to preferred practice pattern, diagnostic classification, and ICD-9-CM codes.
2. Determine appropriate examination process, including tests and measures.
3. Evaluate to determine the appropriate diagnosis, prognosis, and interventions.

The reader should know that the patient was a 32-year-old male who was otherwise healthy. On awakening, he noticed drooping of the right corner of his mouth and an inability to completely close his right eye. He later noted an inability to keep food in the mouth when eating. Later that day, he visited his physician, who made the diagnosis of Bell's palsy. The physician prescribed oral corticosteroids for 1 week (with gradual discontinuation during the second week) and an eye patch and referred the patient for physical therapy. The patient arrived for the first physical therapy visit 1 day after onset with a referral that read "Bell's palsy—right. Evaluate and treat."

What components should the physical therapist incorporate into the examination process (including tests and measures)?

The referring physician gave the diagnosis as Bell's palsy. The physical therapist should complete a patient history and systems review to learn about issues that may influence the plan of care. For example, a history of cardiac arrhythmias may preclude the use of electric stimulation devices as an intervention. The therapist uses the information obtained from the history and systems review to screen for undiagnosed problems that may require further evaluation by the referring physician or other health care practitioner.

For a patient with Bell's palsy, the therapist should conduct a detailed examination of facial musculature and cranial nerve VII function. This examination might include the following components: muscle strength, power, and endurance during functional activities; electroneuromyography; strength-duration testing; and reaction to degeneration testing.

Examination

HISTORY

The patient, a high school English teacher, reported several bouts of low back pain in the past that had resolved with modification of activities for several days. He reported no significant health problems. He did not use tobacco, and he consumed alcohol only occasionally.

SYSTEMS REVIEW

The systems review yielded no signs of undetected health problems.

TESTS AND MEASURES

The patient was unable to voluntarily contract any of the muscles innervated by the right cranial nerve VII. He could not close the right eye voluntarily, and saliva drooled from the right corner of his mouth. The therapist was able to produce strong twitch and tetanic contractions in the muscles innervated by the right cranial nerve VII using pulsatile current. The stimulation parameters were biphasic, asymmetric, balanced pulses; 300 μsec initial negative phase duration and 1200 μsec positive phase duration; no interval between phases; 30 Hz and amplitude 1.5 mA (Figure 8-1). Contractions of similar quality

31

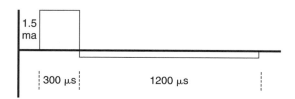

FIGURE 8-1 Biphasic, asymmetric, balanced pulse.

and strength could be produced on the left (unaffected) side using the same pulse characteristics.

A 1-cm-diameter handheld electrode was used to apply current to the seventh cranial nerve and the involved muscles, and a 10-cm × 10-cm electrode was applied to the right arm. The therapist was able to produce twitch contractions in the muscles innervated by cranial nerve VII bilaterally using direct current. Twitch contractions were observed when the cathode was applied to the muscle motor points and when the tap-key of the hand-held electrode was closed.

Evaluation

The ability to induce tetanic contractions with pulsed current and twitch contractions with sudden-onset cathodal direct current indicated that Wallerian degeneration had not taken place. Because there was no trauma, and considering the medical diagnosis (Bell's palsy), it seemed likely that the patient had sustained either a first-degree (neurapraxia) or second-degree injury to cranial nerve VII.[1] Presumably, Bell's palsy is due to compression and ischemia of cranial nerve VII as it courses through the temporal bone. This may be due to swelling associated with immune or viral disease.[2]

Diagnosis

Physical Therapist Practice Pattern 5D: Impaired Motor Function and Sensory Integrity Associated With Nonprogressive Disorders of the Central Nervous System— Acquired in Adolescence or Adulthood.

What is the expected natural course of recovery for this patient?

Prognosis (including plan of care)

If the patient had sustained a first-degree injury, then conduction distal to the injury site would be preserved, and recovery would be expected within a few weeks of onset. If he had sustained a second-degree injury, then the prognosis for recovery would remain good. Axon regeneration would be expected to occur at a rate of about 1 to 2 mm per day.[1]

Electrodiagnostic testing (i.e., nerve conduction velocity testing) may aid in formulating a more accurate prognosis. If Wallerian degeneration had occurred, then signs of gradual denervation would become evident during the 21-day period after the initial onset of symptoms. Signs of denervation that the therapist could elicit would include decreasing response to increasing amplitudes of pulsatile current and a slow, wormlike response to direct current.

SHORT-TERM GOALS

Goals for this patient included restoring muscle performance (i.e., strength, power, endurance) and the ability to perform physical actions, tasks, and activities related to self-care.[3] The timeline for achieving these goals was 8 weeks. The plan included five visits during the first week, then reevaluation of visit frequency at the beginning of the second week. Based on the identified preferred practice pattern, ICD-9-CM code 351.0 was selected for billing purposes.

Intervention

Pulsatile current, with pulse characteristics as noted earlier, was used daily for the first week of treatment. A total of 20 contractions were elicited in each of the affected muscles. The patient was taught how to perform massage to the affected muscles and how to attempt voluntary muscle contractions using a mirror for feedback.[4] At 1 week after onset, obvious signs of denervation were present, and the therapist added direct current to the treatment regimen. At 3 weeks after onset, the therapist could no longer elicit contractions using pulsatile current. Direct current was continued, and the patient was instructed in the use of a home stimulator. The patient returned for reevaluation weekly.

Outcome

At 4 weeks after onset, contractions of minimal strength could be elicited by maximum voluntary effort in some of the affected muscles. During the next three weekly visits, the patient exhibited increasingly stronger voluntary contractions in increasingly more of the affected muscles. By 8 weeks after onset, muscle strength improved to "fair" (i.e., complete range of motion against gravity), and electric stimulation was discontinued. The patient was able to consistently close his right eye and no longer experienced drooling from the right corner of his mouth. Because the goals had been met, physical therapy was discontinued. A follow-up visit was scheduled for 6 months after onset. At the 6-month follow-up visit, muscle strength had improved to "normal" (i.e., complete range of motion against strong pressure). The patient was satisfied with the outcome and noted no continuing impairments, functional limitations, or disabilities.

Discussion

Evidence for the efficacy of electric stimulation in treating Bell's palsy is ambiguous. Ysunza et al[5] studied the use of electric stimulation in patients who underwent nerve grafting after facial palsy and concluded that electric stimulation induced improvement. Targan et al[6] studied the effect of electric stimulation on two groups of patients with chronic facial nerve palsy, one group with idiopathic Bell's palsy and the other group

with acoustic neuroma excision, and concluded that long-term electrical stimulation may facilitate partial reinnervation. It is worthwhile to note that stimulation was kept at submotor levels for this study. Jaweed[1] has indicated that excessive physical or electrical activity during reinnervation may have deleterious effects.

Given the ambiguity of the evidence, it seemed prudent to use motor-level electric stimulation in an attempt to maintain muscle contractibility while denervation, and then reinnervation occurred. The therapist chose to induce 20 contractions of moderate strength daily, hoping that this regimen would not constitute excessive activity. Massage was used to maintain flexibility and perhaps increase circulation in the affected muscles. The therapist believed that voluntary effort with mirror feedback served to promote muscle reeducation.

REFERENCES

1. Jaweed MM: Peripheral nerve regeneration. In Downey JA *et al* (eds): *The physiological basis of rehabilitation medicine* (ed 2), Boston: Butterworth-Heinemann, 1994.
2. Beers M, Berkow R (eds): *The Merck manual of diagnosis and therapy* (ed 17), Whitehouse Station, NJ: Merck & Co, 1999.
3. American Physical Therapy Association: Guide to physical therapist practice, second edition, *Phys Ther* 81:9, 2001.
4. Ross B, Nedzelski JM, McLean A: Efficacy of feedback training in long-standing facial nerve paresis, *Laryngoscope* 101:744, 1991.
5. Ysunza A, Inigo F, Oritz-Monasterio F, *et al*: Recovery of congenital facial palsy in patients with hemifacial mocrosomia subjected to sural to facial nerve grafts is enhanced by electric field stimulation. *Arch Med Res* 27:7, 1996.
6. Targan RS, Alon G, Kay SL: Effect of long-term electrical stimulation on motor recovery and improvement of clinical residuals in patients with unresolved facial nerve palsy, *Otolaryngol Head Neck Surg* 122:246, 2000.

LEARNING OBJECTIVES

The reader will be able to:

1. Analyze the importance of a training schedule.
2. Differentiate between a bone scan and a radiograph.
3. Compare the physiological effects produced by aquatic, closed-chain, and open-chain exercises.

The reader should know that a young woman arrived at an outpatient facility. As the therapist reviewed the intake form, it was noted that the patient was 15 years old, and it was evident that her parents or coach were not present. She reported that a friend drove her to the appointment. Because parental consent was required for the therapist to examine and treat a minor, the appointment was rescheduled for the next evening.

When the parents were present, the therapist inquired if they had brought a prescription. The patient replied that she did not have one, that her coach had referred her to the clinic. The patient's father added that it was extremely important that his daughter be able to return to competition as soon as possible, because they were hopeful that she would receive a college cross-country scholarship.

The patient reported that her hip pain started about 2½ weeks earlier. She described the pain as "sharp" and "shooting," in the right anterior thigh. Initially, it occurred after a few miles of running, but worsened to the point of hurting when walking or climbing steps.

The patient reported that cross-country season had started 4 weeks earlier, and that she had done no training in the off-season. The team ran 6 days a week; the runners did not stretch before or after running and did no supplemental weight training. The coach had them performing walking lunges around the track at school. She had not recently changed her footwear for running. The team trained on a combination of sidewalks and roadways.

The patient denied any relevant past medical history except for exercise-induced asthma. She was taking no medications nor applying any heat or ice to the area of injury. She also denied any changes in her menstrual cycle.

Examination and Evaluation

Physical examination revealed the following findings:

- Strength MMT: Right quadriceps, 4/5; right adductor and hamstring, 4+/5; right hip external rotators, 4/5; right hip abductors, 3+/5; all of the foregoing for the left side, 5/5.
- Sensation: Intact to light touch bilateral lower extremities.
- Posture: Increased lumbar lordosis, genu recurvatum.
- Balance: Unilateral stance with eyes open: right decreased compared with left secondary to pain.
- Squat test: Patient weight shifted to left during the flexion component of the squat. Single leg squat: right, 20 degrees of knee flexion; left, 60 degrees of knee flexion.
- Gait analysis: Positive Trendelenberg's sign, hyperpronation right greater than left at midstance.
- Biomechanical: Right Q-angle 20 degrees, Left Q-angle 18 degrees; leg lengths even; moderate forefoot varus, R>L; bilateral increased external tibia torsion
- Arch height: Normal non–weight bearing, decreased in weight bearing.
- Range of motion: Spine and lower extremity WFL
- Special tests: Negative Thomas, Faber, and Ober tests.

- Lumbar spine: Negative for SLR and slump test.
- Flexibility: Moderate restrictions bilateral calf, quadricep, hamstring, and piriformis.
- Palpation: No palpable tenderness in the hip or lumbar spine.
- Running shoes: More than 1 year old, slip last, semicurved shoe with worn-out heel counter.

Diagnosis

Physical Therapist Practice Pattern 4E: Impaired Joint Mobility, Motor Function, Muscle Performance, and Range of Motion Associated With Localized Inflammation.

What information did the squat test provide?

The unilateral squat test demonstrated the patient's ability to eccentrically control knee flexion (Figure 9-1). It can demonstrate

abnormal biomechanics and weakness of the hip, knee, or ankle musculature. This is a sport-specific skill that is needed during the shock-absorption phase of running.

What features should the patient's running shoes have had, based on her foot type?

The desired shoe features for a patient who pronates are a straight last, board construction, and a strong heel counter with less than 300 miles of wear.

What type of progressive intervention could be used to return this patient to cross-country running?

The early stages concentrated on cross-training to maintain endurance. This was accomplished with a bicycle and aqua jogger. Improving lower extremity flexibility was also important. Non–weight-bearing exercises were progressed to weight-bearing strengthen-

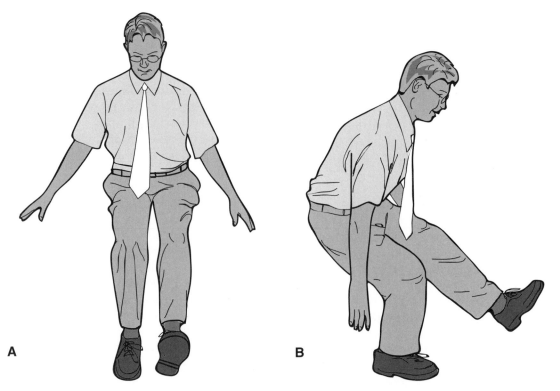

FIGURE 9-1 Single-leg squat. **A,** Front view. **B,** Side view.

ing, focusing on the eccentric gluteus medius, piriformis, quadriceps, and posterior tibialis. Closed-chain exercises, (e.g., step-downs and squats) were then progressed to jumping in a step-jump-hop progression. Once this was accomplished, an interval-jogging program was instituted.

Intervention

WEEK 1

The patient was referred to medical imaging; plain film radiographs were negative. The patient began her physical therapy treatment with a 10-minute warm-up on an exercise bike, followed by stretching of the piriformis, quadriceps, hamstring, and calves. Application of ice concluded the treatment. The therapist noted a decrease in Trendelenburg's sign with the warm-up, but the patient still reported pain on ambulation.

WEEK 2

The patient began by continuing with the previous treatment, then added non–weight-bearing strengthening exercises, including four-way straight-leg raises, prone hamstring curls, external hip rotation with tubing for resistance, and ankle inversion with a theraband.

The patient reported decreased pain after exercising, but no change in the symptoms at school. She was referred to an orthopedic physician with a recommendation to use crutches to ambulate and a request for a bone scan.

What were the advantages of a bone scan versus a plain film radiograph in this case?

The main advantages of a bone scan are the early detection of and increased sensitivity for detecting bone fractures.

WEEK 3

The bone scan revealed periostitis of the femur. The physician wanted to continue physical therapy with a non–weight-bearing program with increased time on the exercise bike and the addition of a home aquatic exercise program with the aqua jogger.

What was the goal of increasing the time on the bike or the aqua jogger?

The goal of increasing the time on the bike or aqua jogger was to improve and maintain the patient's cardiovascular fitness.

WEEKS 4 TO 7

Physical therapy was continued with a non–weight-bearing program, increasing the time on the bike and adding a home exercise program with an aqua jogger. At the end of the fourth week, the patient's pain on walking resolved.

WEEKS 8 TO 11

Weight-bearing exercises were gradually added, with a slow progression of the following: wall sits, step-ups, single-leg balance, leg press, BAPS board, closed chain supination/pronation in ankle plantar flexion, lower extremity exercises, step-downs, plyo-ball toss, and resisted gait. At the end of the eleventh week, Trendelenburg's sign resolved.

Outcome

A running analysis revealed a greater amount of pronation than during ambulation. The patient was advised to purchase Spenco over-the-counter orthotics. A return to a running program was initiated. This included a bike warm-up, stretching, and mini-trampoline jogging every other day, increasing the time from 5, to 7, to 9, to 11 minutes.

The patient progressed to a treadmill for a 2-minute walk, a 5-minute run, and a 2-minute walk. She continued with the walk-run-walk combination every other day, progressing to 5-, 7-, 7-, 10-, 10-, 14-, 14-, 20-, and 20-minute runs. The patient was discharged at the 10-minute run and was to continue the program on her own. At that time, the cross-country season was over.

What was the benefit of having the patient jog on the mini-trampoline before running on the treadmill or sidewalk?

The main benefit of jogging on the mini-trampoline was the decreased impact forces. In this case the athlete had an overuse injury with weight bearing.

Why did the therapist wait until the twelfth week to start the patient jogging?

Certain progressive criteria needed to be met before the patient could return to sports activities. The patient needed to demonstrate pain-free ambulation, a 45-degree unilateral squat with good biomechanics, and the ability to perform 25 unilateral heel raises.

RECOMMENDED READINGS

O'Kane JW: Anterior hip pain, *Am Fam Physician* 60:1687, 1999.

Steele PM: Management of acute fractures around the knee, ankle and foot, *Clin Fam Pract* 2:661, 2000

Alonso JE, Lee J, Burgess AR et al: The management of complex orthopedic injuries, *Surg Clin North Am* 76:879, 1996.

Eiff PM, Hatch RL, Walter CL: *Fracture management for primary care*, Philadelphia: WB Saunders, 1998.

Greenspan A: *Orthopedic radiology* (ed 2), New York: Raven Press, 1992.

Kaufman D, Leung J: Evaluation of the patient with extremity trauma: An evidence-based approach, *Emerg Med Clin North Am* 17:77, 1999.

Shamus E, Shamus J: *Sports injury prevention and rehabilitation*, New York: McGraw-Hill, 2001.

LEARNING OBJECTIVES

The reader will be able to:

1. Differentiate between work hardening and work conditioning.
2. Compare the different levels of duty and lifting restrictions.
3. Apply biomechanical factors to designing a desk workstation.
4. Define the Occupational Safety and Health Administration (OSHA) and Americans With Disability Act (ADA) guidelines.

The reader should know that a physical therapist established a new ergonomic contract with a large electronics production facility. The facility had more than 200 employees with many different job descriptions and physical demands. Some employees needed to carry boxes, whereas others had desk jobs.
The therapist was to develop an injury prevention program, a prescreening program, and education classes. In addition, the chief executive officer (CEO) wanted her workstation assessed.

Diagnosis

Guide to Physical Therapist Practice, Procedural Interventions, p. S108: Functional Training in Work (Job/School/Play), Community, and Leisure Integration or Reintegration (Including Instrumental Activities of Daily Living, Work Hardening, and Work Conditioning).

Intervention

What were important sources of information that the therapist used to help fulfill contractual obligations?

The physical therapist obtained copies of OSHA and ADA guidelines for review.

What was the main component of each guideline?

OSHA: Each employer must furnish employees employment free from recognized hazards that are causing or likely to cause death or physical harm.

ADA: Main guidelines for developing job descriptions; requisite skills; essential job functions, and manner by which job is performed.

After reviewing all of the guidelines, the therapist performed a job/work risk analysis for one of the stock employees. The work analysis consisted of analyzing the employee's job duties by observing the employee performing the essential duties of the job function. This analysis included, but was not limited to, posture, biomechanics, forces, temperature, vibration, repetitions, and pacing. It was important to also look at the floor, equipment, workstation, and office environment. During the analysis, the therapist noticed that the employee had to repetitively lift 40-pound boxes to a height of 4 feet, and that the employee did not have good lifting mechanics. The recommendation to the supervisor was to train the employee in lifting mechanics and also to provide the employee with a hydraulic lift.

This process was repeated for all of the employees. Adapting the tasks, workstation, tools and equipment reduced physical stresses, which helped decrease musculoskeletal disorders.

The next step was to design the CEO's workstation. The CEO spent most of her day sitting behind the desk working on the computer.

What were important areas to consider when setting up a desk workstation?

These areas included seat height, seat back angle, knee and ankle angle, back height and support, elbow alignment, wrist angle, table height, knee clearance, keyboard height, screen height, viewing angle and distance, keyboard and mouse design, screen glare, and room lighting. One factor that required changing was the oversized leather chair. It was not suitable for proper body support while working on the computer, so a new ergonomic computer chair was ordered.

What were the benefits of physical therapy intervention to the workers and the company?

When all of the jobs were analyzed, proper equipment was obtained, and the setup was corrected, it was time to complete the injury prevention program. All employees received education in biomechanics of lifting and fitness evaluations of strength, flexibility, and cardiac condition based on their job duties. Individualized programs were established. Educational classes were also implemented for nutrition, walking, flexibility, body mechanics, and other topics as needed. Many companies have realized decreased medical costs and decreased lost time from work by implementing various types of wellness programs.

Before the therapist secured the contract with the company, one employee working in the packaging area sustained a back injury and was placed on light duty.

What are the different levels of duty and lifting restrictions?

According to the Department of Labor and the Social Security Administration, all jobs fit into one of five levels of exertion: sedentary work, light work, medium work, heavy work, or very heavy work. Jobs are also classified into one of three skill levels: unskilled, semiskilled, and skilled. The National Institute for Occupational Safety and Health has published guidelines for ergonomic manual lifting.

The employee who sustained a back injury was referred to the therapist for rehabilitation. The referring physician requested physical therapy intervention, specifically work-hardening and work-conditioning programs.

What is the difference between work hardening and work conditioning?

Work conditioning usually involves one or two disciplines, comprises primarily exercise and education, takes 2 to 4 hours per day, and usually lasts up to 6 weeks. Work hardening is a more complex program that involves at least several disciplines, uses work simulation as a primary source of treatment in conjunction with exercise and education, takes 2 to 8 hours per day, and typically lasts for 6 to 8 weeks. Once the employee completed the work-conditioning and then the work-hardening programs, the employer wanted to know whether the employee was ready to return to full duty. To make this determination, the therapist decided to perform a functional capacity examination (FCE).

What is an FCE?

The therapist reviewed what was already done via the work-hardening/work-conditioning programs. Next, the therapist compared the employee's physical abilities with the physical demands of the job as specified by the U.S. Department of Labor in the U.S. Department of Transportation (DOT). The FCE was then performed using visual and objective measurements, as well as physiological measurements of heart rate and blood pressure. Some of the categories performed during the FCE were lift, carry, push/pull, elevated work, lowered or forward work, unweighted rotation, crawl, kneel, sustained crouch, repetitive squat, stair ambulation, balance and stabilization, sitting, and upper extremity coordination. The employee's self-reported assessments (e.g., pain, fatigue) were also obtained. It is important to remember that prevention of injury to the employee (i.e., safety) was the first concern.

Outcome

The employee was able to perform all of her job duties without complaints and with proper body mechanics. She returned to full-time duty without restrictions.

RECOMMENDED READINGS

U.S. Department of Labor, Bureau of Labor Statistics: News release: Lost work-time injuries and illnesses; characteristics and resulting time away from work, 1998. April 20, 2000.

National Institute for Occupational Safety and Health: *Work practices guide for manual lifting* (pub 81-122), Cincinnati, Ohio: US Public Health Service, 1981.

Bunn III W: Health, safety, and productivity in a manufacturing environment, *J Occup Environ Med* 43:47, 2001.

King PM: A critical review of functional capacity evaluations, *Phys Ther* 78:852, 1998.

Harten JA: Functional capacity evaluation, *Occup Med* 13:209, 1998.

Isernhagen SJ: *Work injury*, Gaithersburg, Maryland: Aspen, 1988.

Towers Perrin: *Regaining control of workers' compensation costs: the second biennial Towers Perrin survey report*, New York: Towers Perrin, 1994.

Association for Worksite Health Promotion, US Department of Health and Human Services, William M. Mercer, Inc: *1999 national worksite health promotion survey*, Northbrook, Illinois: Association for Worksite Health Promotion and William M. Mercer, Inc, 2000.

Woo M, Yap AK, Oh TG, Long FY: The relationship between stress and absenteeism, *Singapore Med J* 40:1, 1999.

Lechner L, deVries H, Adriaansen S, Drabbels L: Effects of an employee fitness program on reduced absenteeism, *J Occup Environ Med* 39:827, 1997.

Mobley EM, Linz DH, Shukla R, et al: Disability case management: an impact assessment in an automotive manufacturing organization, *J Occup Environ Med* 42:597, 2000.

Rubens AJ, Oleckno WA, Papaeliou L: Establishing guidelines for the identification of occupational injuries: a systematic appraisal, *J Occup Environ Med* 37:151, 1995.

Wyman DO: Evaluating patients for return to work, *Am Fam Physician* 59:844, 1999.

US Department of Labor, Bureau of Labor Statistics: *Workplace injuries and illnesses in 1995* (pub 97-76), Washington, DC: US Government Printing Office, 1997.

National Safety Council: *Accident facts*, Itasca, Illinois: National Safety Council, 1997.

Schibanoff J (ed): *Workers' compensation: health care management guidelines*, vol 7, Washington, DC: Milliman and Robertson, 1998.

LEARNING OBJECTIVES

The reader will be able to:

1. Analyze the role of the sesamoid and flexor hallicus longus (FHL) muscles.
2. Analyze the progression of return to sport activities.
3. Explain the biomechanical role of the foot intrinsic muscles.

The reader should know that a 19-year-old male college football player presented with complaints of pain in the right great toe with walking. He had stopped playing football a year earlier because of the inability to run and cut. He remembered injuring the toe last football season but did not receive any formal treatment at that time. He applied ice for a few days and had hoped the pain would go away once football season was over. Football practice was scheduled to restart in 1 month, and he was frustrated that the right great toe pain persisted. The patient denied any previous lower extremity injuries, and there was nothing significant in the past medical history. He had recently visited a podiatrist, who examined the foot. Radiographs were negative for fracture of bipartite sesamoids. The patient was referred to physical therapy with a diagnosis of sesamoiditis. The physician was optimistic that no surgery would be required. The patient was not taking any medication currently.

What are the roles of the sesamoid bones?

The sesamoids act as mechanical "pulleys" to allow for force generation. They allow for distribution of force and provide a mechanical advantage. Another example of a sesamoid is the patella.

What is a bipartite sesamoid?

A sesamoid is called *bipartite* if the bone did not completely ossify and there can be two pieces instead of one (Figure 11-1).

Will a radiograph always detect a fracture?

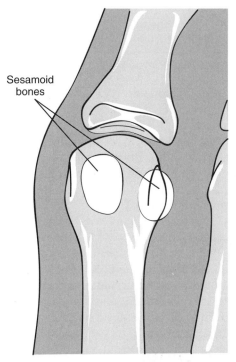

Sesamoid bones

FIGURE 11-1 Bipartite sesamoid.

A radiograph will not always detect a fracture. Depending on the view and osteoblast calcification, a bone scan may be more effective.

Examination and Evaluation

PASSIVE RANGE OF MOTION

Mobility testing (Table 11-1) revealed capsular tightness in the first metacarpophalangeal joint (MPJ) and decreased sesamoid mobility along with decreased flexibility in hamstrings and piriformis bilaterally, and the

43

TABLE 11-1
MOBILITY/STRENGTH DATA

DEGREES	R	L
Dorsiflexion	3	12
Plantarflexion	50	50
First MPJ extension	35	85

MANUAL MUSCLE TEST

	R	L
DF	5	5
INV	5	5
EV	4+	5
First MPJ extension	4+	5
Hip and knee	5	5

MPJ, Metacarpophalangeal joint.

right gastrocnemius. Gait analysis revealed decreased heel raise and push off on the right foot.

Single-leg balance on the right extremity was 30 seconds with the patient's eyes open and 3 seconds with the eyes closed. Arch heights, both weight bearing and non-weight bearing, were normal.

Diagnosis

Guide to Physical Therapist Practice Pattern 4E: Impaired Joint Mobility, Motor Function, Muscle Performance, and Range of Motion Associated With Localized Inflammation.

Intervention

The patient began with 7 minutes on the exercise bike to begin to increase blood flow and pliability of the musculature and soft tissue. This was followed by bilateral stretching of the calf, hamstring, and piriformis muscles for 3 × 30 seconds. Pulsed ultrasound was applied to the plantar aspect of the great toe, followed by first MPJ Maitland mobilization grade III and IV dorsal glides/distraction and sesamoid grade III mobilization superior and inferior to decrease pain and inflammation and increase A/PROM, joint mobility, and flexibility. As A/PROM increased, neuromuscular retraining and strengthening was initiated, with seated heel raises for toe exten-

sion (30 repetitions), towel crunches with a 2-pound weight, and isometric first MPJ flexion (10 × 10 seconds), with no flexion of the interphalangeal joint permitted. Ankle eversion strengthening was progressed to theraband therapy. Proprioception exercises included single-leg balance with eyes closed, gait training for extension and first metatarsal stabilization, and resisted gait in all planes with single-leg balance at the end position. After exercise, ice and electric stimulation were used to decrease pain and inflammation.

As range of motion and strength were restored, the patient was progressed to sport-specific running and agility drills.

Outcome

The patient had an excellent outcome. He was able to increase his 40-yard dash time by 4/10 of a second and return to playing football. The patient continues with ongoing intrinsic stabilization and strengthening of the FHL muscle.

REFERENCES

1. Adelaar RS: *Disorders of the great toe.* Rosemont, Illinois: American Academy of Orthopedic Surgeons, 1997.
2. Aper RL, Saltzman CL, Brown TD: The effect of hallux sesamoid excision on the flexor hallucis longus moment arm, *Clin Orthop* 325:209, 1996.
3. Aper RL, Saltzman CL, Brown TD: The effect of hallux sesamoid resection on the effective moment of the flexor hallucis brevis, *Foot Ankle Int* 15:462, 1994.
4. Aseyo D, Nathan H: Hallux sesamoid bones: anatomical observations with special reference to osteoarthritis and hallux valgus, *Int Orthop* 8:67, 1984.
5. Baechle TR (ed): *Essentials of strength training and conditioning,* ed 2, Champaign, Illinois, 2001, Human Kinetics.
6. Battista J: Pro football Testaverde may start against Giants despite toe injury. *New York Times* August, 17:1, 2000.
7. Boissonnault W, Donatelli R: The influence of hallux extension on the foot during ambulation, *J Orthop Sports Phys Ther* 5:240, 1984.

8. Camasta CA: Hallux limitus and hallux rigidus: clinical examination, radiographic findings and natural history, *Clin Podiatr Med Surg* 13:423, 1996.
9. Canavan PK: *Rehabilitation in sports medicine: a comprehensive guide*, Stamford, Conn, 1998, Appleton and Lange.
10. Churchill RS, Donley BG: Managing injuries of the great toe, *Phys Sports Med* 26:1, 1998.
11. Clanton TO, Ford JJ: Turf toe injury, *Clin Sports Med* 13:731, 1994.
12. Clanton TO, Butler JE, Eggert A: Injuries to the metatarsophalangeal joints in athletes, *Foot Ankle* 7:162, 1986.
13. Cohn I, Kanat IO: Functional limitations of motion of the first metatarsophalangeal joint, *J Foot Surg* 23:477, 1984.
14. Coker TP, Arnold JA. Weber DL: Traumatic lesions of the metatarsophalangeal joint of the great toe in athletes, *Am J Sports Med* 6:326, 1978.
15. Dananberg HJ: Functional hallux limitus and its relationship to gait efficiency, *J Am Podiatr Med Assoc* 76:648, 1986.
16. David RD, Delagoutte JP, Renard MM: Anatomical study of the sesamoid bones of the first metatarsal, *J Am Podiatr Med Assoc* 79:536, 1989.
17. DeLauro TM, Positano RG: Surgical management of hallux limitus and rigidus in the young patient, *Clin Podiatr Med Surg* 6:83, 1989.

LEARNING OBJECTIVES

The reader will be able to:

1. State how knowledge gained in research on constraint-induced movement therapy (CIMT) can be applied in the clinic.
2. Express how application of CIMT was appropriate with a specific patient.
3. Identify how intervention was planned using CIMT research and how objective measures were used to measure the outcomes in a patient.

The reader should know that the parents of a 5-year-old child with hemiplegic spastic cerebral palsy approached their physical therapist about improving their child's upper extremity use. The parents were concerned that their child had more ability to use his upper extremity than he was demonstrating. This child's physical therapist had recently read a research article about learned nonuse and intervention using constraint-induced movement therapy (CIMT) in adults after stroke, and was curious whether this approach would be appropriate for her young patient.

Examination

HISTORY

This 5-year-old boy was the fourth pregnancy and birth for a 32-year-old mother and 30-year-old father. The mother experienced bleeding 36 weeks into her pregnancy. Ultrasonography determined that the baby was in a breech position. The mother and father decided on a cesarean section at 36 weeks secondary to the mother's history of early deliveries and quick labors.

The 4-lb, 2-oz infant was delivered without complications. Immediately after birth, the infant exhibited respiratory problems, and he was transferred to the hospital's neonatal intensive care unit (NICU). In the NICU, the infant received oxygen and was placed on a warming table secondary to problems with thermoregulation. After 2 days in the NICU, the infant was transferred to the newborn nursery; after 5 days, he went home with his parents.

At age 3 years, the child was referred for physical and occupational therapy after a diagnosis of right hemiplegic cerebral palsy. The parents initiated a neurologic examination after the child's second birthday when they became concerned about his asymmetrical gait and lack of right upper extremity use. Just before his third birthday, the child began physical therapy (Figure 12-1), 60-minute sessions twice per week. Approximately 1 month before this initial consultation (nearly 2 years after initiation of therapy), physical therapy was decreased to one 60-minute session per week.

At the time of the initial evaluation to consider CIMT, the parents reported that the child did not spontaneously use his right (involved) upper extremity unless he needed to stabilize an object. The parents felt that the child had the ability to use the upper extremity more during his daily functioning. The physical therapist was not familiar with CIMT and was unsure whether this therapy would benefit this child.

Could CIMT be a useful intervention technique for this child?

The therapist did a literature search on CIMT and found a significant amount of research on CIMT in adults,[1-13] but only limited reports of CIMT in children.[14-16] How could this therapist determine whether this type of treatment would be appropriate for this child?

The therapist needed to answer a few questions:

1. *Was there enough evidence in the literature to suggest that CIMT is an effective*

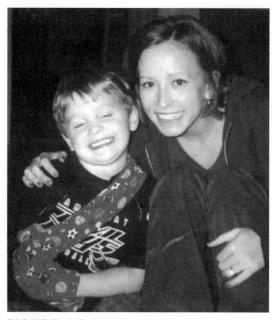

FIGURE 12-1 Child with cerebral palsy, shown with physical therapy student.

treatment? The therapist decided that the evidence in adults was very strong. Although the evidence for CIMT's efficacy in children was not as strong, the therapist decided that it was sufficient to consider CIMT a viable approach for specific children.

2. *Did this child fit the description of subjects who have demonstrated improvements after CIMT intervention?* Most of the research on CIMT has been done on subjects who have had a stroke or on children with hemiplegia.[1-16] The child's diagnosis was consistent with that of pediatric subjects who have used CIMT.[14-16] The therapist decided that the child's diagnosis of hemiplegic cerebral palsy would be appropriate for this intervention method. This child was significantly younger than the adult subjects who had experienced success[1-13]; however, the therapist found some reports on pediatric subjects, ranging in age from 15 months to 13 years.[14-16] The therapist decided the child's age was appropriate for this intervention.

3. *Did this child meet the strict inclusion criteria set forth in the evidence found on CIMT?[1-16]* The therapist determined that the child met all of the following criteria:
   - The child was of normal intelligence.
   - The child was able to extend his wrist 10 degrees and his fingers to neutral.
   - The child did have sensation present in his involved upper extremity, although the therapist surmised that there may have been some decreased sensation based on the child's limited use of the involved upper extremity.
   - The child had sufficient balance to have his uninvolved upper extremity constrained without compromising his safety, and the therapist judged that he would be able to tolerate wearing a sling.
   - The child relied primarily on his uninvolved upper extremity (left upper extremity) for all functional activities. He used his right (involved) upper extremity for weight bearing and if asked to use it, but the parents reported that he needed to be reminded to use it.
   - The parents were agreeable to the intervention, understood the time required for carryover at home, and were realistic about the possible outcomes.

   Based on this information, the therapist decided the child would be an appropriate candidate for CIMT intervention. The therapist then needed to find the space and a therapist or team of therapists to provide this intensive intervention. The therapist enlisted the help of a local physical therapist education program. The program provided space and physical therapy students to carry out the intervention. A research review board at the local physical therapy education program approved the intervention.

4. *How was the intervention carried out?* Research on CIMT has focused on long daily periods of intervention for an intense period.[4] The intervention has used shaping, defined as providing enough assistance to ensure success while encouraging the

subject to do as much as he or she can.[4] In addition, constraint of the uninvolved upper extremity for 90% of waking hours has been provided to ensure that the involved upper extremity is used. CIMT has emphasized functional intervention.[4] The therapist and the parents determined a list of functions they wanted to improve with the child's right (involved) upper extremity. These included tooth brushing, hair combing, eating with a fork/spoon, picking up food, playing with toys, and throwing a ball with the father and older siblings.

Evaluation

Based on an examination of the child, the therapist concluded that there were three major inhibitors to the child using his right upper extremity: (1) poor coordination between the fingers and thumb, (2) learned nonuse, and (3) decreased hand strength. During function, the child demonstrated poor coordination between his fingers and poor ability to prepare his hand for and grip objects. Throughout his life, the child had learned that his left upper extremity worked more efficiently, and consequently he chose to use the left upper extremity more. Thus, he had learned not to use the involved upper extremity. The therapist concluded that forcing the child to use the right upper extremity would change the habit of using the left upper extremity exclusively. The therapist also concluded that poor strength interfered with the child's ability to successfully grip and manipulate objects. The therapist chose intervention that emphasized gripping a variety of objects and repeated use of hand function to address the poor coordination, learned nonuse, and decreased hand strength.

Diagnosis

Physical Therapist Practice Pattern 5C: Impaired Motor Function and Sensory Integrity Associated With Nonprogressive Disorders of the Central Nervous System—Congenital Origin or Acquired in Infancy or Childhood.

Prognosis (including Plan of Care)

The therapist used the following tests to measure the child's abilities and improvement after the intervention. These tests were chosen because they were all objectively measurable and related to the functions in which the parents wanted to see improvement:

- Spoon transfer of cereal from one bowl to another bowl in 30 seconds.
- Picking up cereal from a tabletop and placing them in a jar with a 1.5-inch diameter opening in 30 seconds.
- Throwing a ball, with the maximum distance and accuracy of the throw measured (when playing catch with family members).
- Stacking 1-inch blocks.
- Picking up quarters from a tabletop and placing them in a coin bank placed at shoulder height in 30 seconds.
- Picking up cards from a tabletop and turning them over in 30 seconds.
- Evaluating grip and pincher strength with a dynamometer.
- Having the parents use a motor log (based on the Pediatric Evaluation of Disability Inventory[17]) to monitor changes at home.

In an effort to gain accurate baseline measures, the child was assessed on these measures three times a week for 2 weeks before initiating the intervention. After these baseline measurements were obtained, the child was seen for intensive intervention 4 hours a day, 5 days a week for 2 weeks.

Intervention

During the time spent in intervention, the child played with many toys he enjoyed at home (e.g., soft molding clay, building blocks, a memory game with cards, a bean bag toss game), and he performed functional skills (e.g., brushing his teeth/hair, making a sandwich, eating with a spoon/fork, picking up food). Throughout the intervention, minimal assistance was given to allow the child to be successful during functioning. The parents were given training to carry out the intervention at home.

In addition to the daily sessions, the child wore a specially designed sling with a glove over his uninvolved hand and a strap around his waist. The glove was attached to the strap around his waist with Velcro to allow the child to quickly release his hand if necessary for balance. The child wore the sling for the 2-week intervention and then for the following week, because the therapist wanted to ensure continued use of the involved upper extremity.

Reexamination

The improvements seen after the 3 weeks of intervention therapy and sling use are summarized in Table 12-1. After the intervention and sling use, the parents reported a

significant increase in the child's spontaneous use of the involved upper extremity throughout the day. The parents reported that the child's need for verbal cues to use the involved upper extremity was decreased, but did note that the child still relied on his left (uninvolved) extremity for some functional activities.

Outcome

The child demonstrated improvement in most of the outcome measures used. The parents reported an improvement in the child's spontaneous use of the involved upper extremity and a decrease in the amount of verbal cues needed to remind the child to use the involved upper extremity. Three months after the intervention, the child was reassessed on the outcome measures. All of the improvements were maintained. The parents reported that the child continued to use the involved upper extremity during bilateral tasks, but continued to prefer using his uninvolved upper extremity during unilat-eral tasks.

TABLE 12-1
IMPROVEMENTS FOLLOWING INTERVENTION

OBJECTIVE MEASURES	PRETESTING	POSTTESTING
Spoon transfer of cereal	34 to 86 pieces of cereal	107 to 135 pieces of cereal
Picking up cereal and placing in jar	12 to 17 pieces of cereal	28 to 45 pieces of cereal
Ball throw	52-90 in; unable to hit target	77.5-131 in; hit target two out of three attempts
Stacking blocks	8 blocks in 28-31 seconds	10 blocks in 39-41 seconds
Quarters in the bank	4-5 quarters	8-9 quarters
Picking up cards	8-10 cards	12-13 cards
Grip strength	3-4 kg	6 kg
Pincher strength	1-2 kg	2.5-3 kg
Daily log	Did not use right upper extremity	Used upper extremity spontaneously with minimal assistance to independent for brushing teeth/hair, using spoon/fork, and playing with toys

REFERENCES

1. Ostendorf CG, Wolf SL: Effect of forced use of the upper extremity of a hemiplegic patient on changes in function, *Phys Ther* 61:1022, 1981.
2. Taub E, Miller NE, Novack TA, et al: Technique to improve chronic motor deficit after stroke, *Arch Phys Med Rehabil* 74:347, 1993.
3. Russo SG: Hemiplegic upper extremity rehabilitation: a review of the force-used paradigm, *Neurol Rep* 19:17, 1995.
4. Taub E, Crago JE, Uswatte G: Constraint-induced movement therapy: a new approach to treatment in physical rehabilitation, *Rehabil Psychol* 43:152, 1998.
5. Miltner W, Bauder H, Sommer N, et al: Effects of constraint-induced movement therapy on patients with chronic motor deficits after stroke: a replication, *Stroke* 30:586, 1999.
6. Kunkel A, Kopp B, Muller G, et al: Constraint-induced movement therapy for motor recovery in chronic stroke patients, *Arch Phys Med Rehabil* 80:624, 1999.
7. Blanton S, Wolf S: An application of upper-extremity constraint-induced movement therapy in a patient with subacute stroke, *Phys Ther* 79:847, 1999.
8. Van der Lee JH, Wagenaar RC, Lankhorst GJ, et al: Forced use in the upper extremity in chronic stroke patients, *Stroke* 30:2369, 1999.
9. Taub E, Uswatte G, Pidikiti R: Constraint-induced movement therapy: a new family of techniques with broad application to physical rehabilitation. A clinical review, *J Rehabil Res Dev* 36:237, 1999.
10. Taub E: Constraint-induced movement therapy and massed practice, *Stroke* 31:986, 2000.
11. Liepert J, Miltner W, Bauder H, et al: Motor cortex plasticity during constraint-induced movement therapy in stroke patients, *Neurosci Lett* 250:5, 1998.
12. Kopp B, Kunkel A, Muhlnickel W, et al: Plasticity in the motor system related to therapy-induced improvement of movement after stroke, *Neuroreport* 10:807, 1999.
13. Liepert J, Bauder H, Miltner W, et al: Treatment-induced cortical reorganization after stroke in humans, *Stroke* 31:1210, 2000.
14. Yasukawa A: Upper extremity casting: adjunct treatment for a child with cerebral palsy hemiplegia, *Am J Occup Ther* 44:840, 1990.
15. Crocker MD, MacKay-Lions M, McDonnell E: Forced use of the upper extremity in cerebral palsy: a single-case design, *J Occup Ther* 51:824, 1997.
16. Charles J, Lavinder G, Gordon AM: Effects of constraint-induced therapy on hand function in children with hemiplegic cerebral palsy, *Pediatr Phys Ther* 13:68, 2001.
17. Haley SM, Faas RM, Coster WJ, et al: *Pediatric evaluation of disabilities inventory (PEDI)*, Boston: New England Medical Center, 1989.

Case 13

LEARNING OBJECTIVES

The reader will be able to:

1. Describe the consultative role of physical therapy in primary prevention of falls for a community-dwelling older adult.
2. Identify major risk factors for falls in community-dwelling older adults.
3. Determine appropriate examination/screening methods to determine fall risk in a community-based setting.
4. Determine appropriate interventions to reduce or eliminate fall risk factors for a community-dwelling older adult.
5. Discuss the need for follow-up to reexamine and determine outcomes in a community-based setting.

The reader should know that the patient, Mrs. G, was a 73-year-old female who lived alone in a small urban community. She attended a health fair and education program for fall risk reduction sponsored by a local nonprofit organization that serves senior citizens. The program was designed and conducted by a physical therapist. After an explanation of the program, Mrs. G gave informed consent to participate.

Examination

HISTORY

Mrs. G completed an intake form that revealed a fall less than 6 months earlier in which she was not injured, but experienced soreness that lasted a few days. She reported that the fall occurred in her kitchen while she was getting a late-night snack from the refrigerator. On further questioning, she revealed that the kitchen lights were not on (apart from the refrigerator light) and that she was walking with socks, but no shoes, on her feet.

Mrs. G also reported an active lifestyle. She participated in activities such as babysitting, baking, household chores, and bus trips three to four times per week. She ambulated independently without an assistive device. She reported a past medical history of cataracts and the use of eyeglasses. She rated her current health as 7.4 on a 10-cm–long visual analog scale anchored by poor health at one end and excellent health on the other end. Her medications included Micro-K, Antacand, and Ocovite.

SYSTEMS REVIEW

What type of screening is appropriate to identify fall risk for a community-dwelling older adult?

Based on a literature review, risk factors that appear to be the most critical for both falls and injury are (1) history of falls, (2) cognitive impairment, (3) gait and balance disorders, (4) lower extremity dysfunction, (5) use of psychotropic medications, and (6) visual impairment.[1] Because falls are typically multifactorial in nature, instrumentation for screening was selected to address several of these targeted areas.

Cognitive status. Mrs. G's knowledge of fall risk factors was assessed by means of a "fall facts" check-off pretest to determine her baseline.[2] Her level of knowledge was based on her ability to identify intrinsic and extrinsic fall risk factors and appropriate methods to reduce or eliminate fall risk factors from a list of correct and incorrect choices. Mrs. G scored 85% correct.

Mrs. G also completed the activities-specific balance confidence scale to measure her confidence to perform particular activities without losing her balance or becoming unsteady.[3] The scale included 16 items that described common, everyday activities. Mrs. G placed a mark on a 10-cm line anchored with 0% to 100% confidence for performing each item. Her average score was 90.1%.

Neuromuscular. Mrs. G's balance was measured by the multi-directional reach test (MDRT)[4] and the timed-up-and-go test (TUG) test.[5] For the MDRT she stood beside a yardstick, with her feet comfortably apart, and raised her arm to 90 degrees elevation. She then reached as far as possible without taking a step. She performed the reach in four directions: forward, backward, and to each side. The distance from the starting point to the finishing point was recorded by measuring the change in location (in inches) of the fingertips on the yardstick in each direction. This test measured postural stability based on the patient's ability to maintain her center of gravity over her base of support and move toward the limits of stability without falling. Her scores were as follows: forward, 7.4 inches; backward, 9.1 inches; right, 8.1 inches; left, 6.4 inches.

For the TUG test, Mrs. G was seated in a standard-size armchair and asked to stand and walk 3 meters, turn around, and return to sitting. This test was timed (in seconds) from the time her back left the chair until she returned to sitting and her back was again resting on the chair. Her time was 10.4 seconds.

Musculoskeletal. Next, Mrs. G. performed the 30-second chair-stand test[6] to evaluate her gross lower extremity strength. In this test, the patient is seated on a chair positioned against a wall (to prevent it from slipping) and instructed to fold both arms across her chest and place her feet apart to shoulder width, positioned slightly behind her knees in a slightly staggered stance. She was encouraged to stand up completely and sit back down as many times as possible within the 30-second time limit. Mrs. G. scored 14 repetitions.

Diagnosis

Physical Therapist Practice Pattern 5A: Primary Prevention/Risk Reduction for Loss of Balance and Falling.

Prognosis

GOAL

Mrs. G. will reduce 10 or more risk factors for falls through instruction to promote awareness and use of community resources, modification of her environment and lifestyle, and participation in a fitness program.

EXPECTED OUTCOMES

In 3 months:
1. Increased knowledge of intrinsic and extrinsic fall risk factors, as evidenced by a 55 to 10% increase in the "fall facts" check-off score.
2. Improved sense of well being as indicated by a 5% to 10% increase in the activities-specific balance confidence scale score.

In 6 months:
3. Improved safety through reduction of five or more intrinsic and extrinsic (each) fall risk factors.
4. Maintained level of physical fitness and balance through participation in tai chi exercise two to three times per week.

Intervention

What type of intervention should be developed based on evidence in the literature for effective fall risk reduction and prevention for community-dwelling older adults?

Following a review of the literature, the therapist found that the most effective interventions to reduce fall risk included exercise to improve balance and/or strength,[7-11] home environment modifications,[10,11] and patient education.[10,11] However, the subjects, methods, and instrumentation varied widely across studies, making it difficult to compare results and determine the optimum approach. Overall, the most comprehensive programs were multifaceted in nature, addressing both intrinsic and extrinsic risk factors.[10,11] The therapist decided to design a program based on components from successful studies that targeted well elderly in a community-based setting.[7,8,10,11]

EDUCATION

Fall risk reduction program. The educational program was designed to instruct community-dwelling older adults on intrinsic and extrinsic risk factors for falls and on strategies to reduce or eliminate these risks. Participants attended three 1-hour in-service sessions that included education about risk factors and prevention via lecture, group discussion, and group activities. Participants were given checklists of both intrinsic and extrinsic risk factors to perform self-assessments.[1] The program also included practicing strategies to get up from the floor in case of a fall. A provocative video, "Fear of Falling,"[12] was shown during the last educational session; this video portrayed several older adults making changes to reduce fall risks and overcome fear. The in-service sessions were held at a local senior center where the participants sat 5 to 6 persons per table. The program was age-sensitive, based on approaches appropriate for older adults. For example, written materials were in a large, simple font (14-point, Arial rounded) and printed on off-white paper to facilitate reading. The reading level for all printed materials was at or below the seventh-grade level, as determined by a Gunning Fog index below 7.0.[13]

Referral to begin a home exercise program. As part of the fall risk reduction program, the importance of improving or maintaining fitness and balance was emphasized. Mrs. G attended tai chi lessons offered at the senior center as a community resource. The class included instruction in 10 tai chi exercises that required weight shifting, rotation, trunk and extremity movements, and a changing base of support. The lessons were offered for 1 hour during three monthly in-service sessions. Participants were instructed to continue practicing the exercises at home two to three times per week and were given a written and illustrated handout including warm-up/cool-down exercises and the 10 tai chi exercises.

Tracking of follow-up to reduce or eliminate fall risks. During and after completion of the education program, Mrs. G was asked to record any attempt to reduce or eliminate a fall risk factor (e.g., scheduling a doctor's appoint-ment, removing a throw rug, buying new footwear, or changing light bulbs). She was also given an activity calendar on which to record her performance of the tai chi home exercise program. The physical therapist visited the senior center for 3 consecutive months after the education component to track progress on risk factor reduction and to motivate participants.

Reexamination

The screening examinations were repeated after 3 months, when the educational program was completed. Mrs. G's scores are given in Table 13-1.

The follow-up for risk factor reduction was categorized based on whether Mrs. G addressed personal (i.e., intrinsic) risk or environmental (i.e., extrinsic) risk and on whether the change required any cost.[15] Mrs. G reported making a total of 16 changes to reduce or eliminate fall risk factors, as listed in Table 13-2.

The follow-up for home exercise was reported based on Mrs. G's activity calendar. She recorded practicing the exercises at home either one to two or three to four times per week over a 6-month period. At the end of the program, she rated her current health as 8.2 on a 10-cm visual analog scale anchored by poor health at one end and excellent health on the other end.

Outcome

On initial screening, Mrs. G scored within normal limits for all of the cognitive, neuromuscular, and musculoskeletal screening examinations. However, her history revealed a recent fall at home, which signaled a need for prevention. She was encouraged to attend the educational program and begin an exercise program to maintain fitness and balance.[8,16] Mrs. G responded well to the educational program by making 16 changes to reduce fall risks. Most of her changes were to reduce environmental risk factors by performing

TABLE 13-1
SCREENING EXAMINATION DATA

SCREENING	PRETEST SCORE	POSTTEST SCORE	PUBLISHED NORMS
Cognition:			
Fall facts checkoff	(% correct) 85.4%	(% correct) 91.7%	100% indicates all items correct
Activities-specific Balance Confidence (ABC) scale	(average confidence) 91%	(average confidence) 94%	100% indicates complete confidence; highly mobile elderly = 80.9% average[3]
Balance:			
Multidirectional reach Test	(inches)	(inches)	(inches)[4]
Forward	7.4	7.0	8.9 ± 3.3
Backward	9.1	9.2	4.6 ± 3.0
Right	8.1	6.8	6.8 ± 3.0
Left	6.4	5.3	6.6 ± 2.8
Timed-Up-and-Go (TUG)	(seconds) 10.4	(seconds) 9.3	(seconds)[14] 9–15
Strength:			
30-second chair-stand test	(repetitions) 14	(repetitions) 13	(repetitions)[6] 13.1 ± 3.4

TABLE 13-2
CHANGES TO REDUCE OR ELIMINATE ALL RISK FACTORS

RISK FACTOR CATEGORY	NUMBER OF CHANGES
Intrinsic risks	
Personal behavior change/no cost	5
Personal behavior change/with cost	1
Extrinsic risks	
Environmental change/no cost	7
Environmental change/with cost	3

such tasks as eliminating clutter, installing nightlights, and removing throw rugs. In addition, she focused on reducing risk-taking behaviors, such as wearing unsafe footwear and walking in the dark. During the follow-up period, she also adhered to the tai chi exercise program as a personal preference for an enjoyable means to maintain fitness. Subjectively, Mrs. G stated that she enjoyed the program and believed that she was able to make important changes to protect herself from falling. She did not report any falls or near falls during the 6-month period of contact with the physical therapist.

Discussion

When planning a prevention/wellness program, what feasibility and design issues should be addressed?

In a community-based setting, such issues as time, cost, and space are important to consider when selecting tests and measures for a fall risk screening program. More importantly, instruments that have established reliability and validity (especially predictive validity for fall risk) should be selected. Based on the literature, targeted fall risk factors may include gait and balance disorders, lower extremity dysfunction, use of psychotropic medications, and visual impairment.[1] Because falls are typically multifactorial in nature, screening should address a few of these targeted areas. In addition, a survey of environmental/home safety can be accomplished with a checklist.[1,17]

Designing a concise yet effective educational program is a challenge in any setting. The teaching methods must match the needs of the target audience. This program was conducted over a 3-month period to allow for review, follow-up, and repeated contact for motivation of participants. The methods were age sensitive and incorporated the use of social support within the older adult peer group. The program included opportunities for observational learning (e.g., getting up from the floor) and improving self-efficacy by means of self-assessment and tracking changes to reduce risks. Reinforcement was also provided via prizes (e.g., household items) and praise from the physical therapist and peers.[18]

As the profession of physical therapy moves toward more of an emphasis on prevention and wellness, therapists may be involved in designing programs such as this to meet community needs.

REFERENCES

1. Tideiksaar R: *Falling in old age* (ed 2), New York: Springer, 1997.
2. Hakim RM: *A fall risk reduction intervention for community-dwelling older adults*, November 2001, available at http://www.lib.umi.com/dissertations/.
3. Powell LE, Myers AM: The activities-specific balance confidence (ABC) scale, *J Gerontol A Biol Sci Med Sci* 50:28, 1995.
4. Newton RA: Multi-directional reach test: a practical measure for limits of stability in older adults, *J Gerontol A Biol Sci Med Sci* 56:1, 2001.
5. Podsiadlo D, Richardson S: The timed up & go: a test of basic functional mobility for frail elderly persons, *J Am Geriatr Soc* 39:142, 1991.
6. Jones JC, Rikli RE, Beam WC: A 30-s chair-stand test as a measure of lower body strength in community-residing older adults, *Res Q Ex Sport* 70:113, 1999.
7. Shumway-Cook A, Gruber W, Baldwin M, Shiquan L: The effect of multidimensional exercises on balance, mobility, and fall risk in community-dwelling older adults, *Phys Ther* 77:46, 1997.
8. Wolf SL, Barnhart HX, Kutner NG, et al: Reducing frailty and falls in older persons: an investigation of tai chi and computerized balance training, *J Am Geriatr Soc* 44:489, 1996.
9. Campbell AJ, Robertson MC, et al: Randomised controlled trial of a general practice program of home based exercise to prevent falls in elderly women, *BMJ* 315:1065, 1997.
10. Tinetti ME, Baker DI, McAvay G, et al: A multi-factorial intervention to reduce the risk of falling among elderly people living in the community, *N Engl J Med* 331:821, 1994.
11. Close J, Ellis M, Hooper R, et al: Prevention of falls in the elderly trial (PROFET): a randomized controlled trial, *Lancet* 353:93, 1999.
12. *Fear of falling*, Watertown, MA: New England Research Institutes (NERI) Media Development Center.
13. The Training Post: *The Gunning Fog index*, available at http://www.trainingpost.org/3-2-inst.html.
14. Newton RA: Balance screening of an inner city older adult population, *Arch Phys Med Rehabil* 78:587, 1997.
15. Ryan J, Spellbring AM: Implementing strategies to decrease risk of falls in older women, *J Gerontol Nurs* 22:25, 1996.
16. Wolfson L, Whipple R, Derby C, et al: Balance and strength training in older adults: intervention gains and tai chi maintenance, *J Am Geriatr Soc* 44:498, 1996.
17. Tideiksaar R: Preventing falls: home hazard checklists to help older patients protect themselves, *Geriatrics* 41:26, 1986.
18. Bandura A: *Social foundations of thought and action: a social cognitive theory*, Englewood Cliffs, NJ: Prentice-Hall, 1986.

LEARNING OBJECTIVES

The reader will be able to:

1. Identify the clinical signs and symptoms presented with poikilothermia.
2. Describe the pathophysiology related to poikilothermia with spinal cord injury patients.
3. Discuss the appropriate physical therapy interventions to prevent poikilothermia.

The reader should know that the patient was a 32-year-old, married, African-American male who sustained a spinal cord injury after a bicycle accident 1 month earlier while riding to his industrial job. Radiographs revealed a C7-T1 fracture dislocation of C7 and severe subluxation (90%) anteriorly on T1. Surgical procedures included stabilization and fusion both anteriorly and posteriorly at these spinal levels. The patient was transferred to a facility 1 month later for rehabilitation, with an examination consistent with C7 ASIA level A quadriparesis (Table 14-1).

On physical therapy examination, the patient had an unremarkable past medical history with no abuse of drugs or alcohol and was functionally independent before his accident. The patient was to wear a Miami-J collar and abdominal binder when out of bed, in addition to compression stockings and bilateral pressure-relief ankle-foot orthoses (PRAFO).

During the initial physical therapy sessions, interventions focused on wheelchair mobility using a manual chair, transfers with the use of a sliding board, upper extremity supported sitting balance, bed mobility, increasing tolerance to vertical positioning with the use of the tilt table, and patient education. The patient made only minimal improvements in all aspects of therapy during the initial 2 weeks, despite his high motivational level. Further progress was limited because of the patient's persistent low-grade fever since admission. The patient also displayed occasional increased perspiration in areas of his face and neck. Many physical therapy sessions had been terminated prematurely secondary to these issues.

TABLE 14-1
ASIA IMPAIRMENT SCALE

ASIA IMPAIRMENT SCALE
☐ **A** = **Complete:** No motor or sensory function is preserved in the sacral segments S4 to S5.
☐ **B** = **Incomplete:** Sensory but not motor function is preserved below the neurologic level and includes the sacral segments S4 to S5.
☐ **C** = **Incomplete:** Motor function is preserved below the neurologic level, and more than half of key muscles below the neurologic level have a muscle grade less than 3.
☐ **D** = **Incomplete:** Motor function is preserved below the neurologic level, and at least half of key muscles below the neurologic level have a muscle grade of 3 or more.
☐ **E** = **Normal:** motor and sensory functions are normal.

CLINICAL SYNDROMES
☐ Central cord ☐ Brown-Sequard ☐ Anterior cord ☐ Conus medullaris ☐ Cauda equina

From American Spinal Cord Injury Association: International Standards for Neurological and Functional Classification of Spinal Cord Injury, Chicago, 1996, p 26. Used with permission.

There was concern about the patient's medical status and the negative effects on his rehabilitative progress.

What would be the appropriate response in this situation?

Examination and Evaluation

HISTORY

The patient was illiterate and from a very poor socioeconomic background. He was extremely slender and appeared to be malnourished. His medications included Lovenox as a deep-vein thrombosis prophylaxis, Didronel as a prophylaxis to avoid heterotopic ossification, Zosyn as an antibiotic, Ambien for insomnia, Robitussin as a cough expectorant, and Colace as a stool softener.

SYSTEMS REVIEW

The patient presented with decreased air entry in the bilateral lung bases, with no rales, rhonchi, or wheezing auscultated. S1 and S2 heart sounds were noted, but no S3 or S4 sounds were appreciated. There were no clubbing, cyanosis, dermatologic compromise, or edema, and dorsalis pedis pulsations were 2+ bilaterally. His vital signs in a seated position revealed a blood pressure of 100/65 mm Hg, respiratory rate of 23 beats per minute (bpm), heart rate of 92 bpm, and temperature of 99.8° C.

TESTS AND MEASURES

Sensation, range of motion, and muscle strength were normal in the preserved levels. Passive range of motion was within normal limits in the involved trunk and lower extremities, and there was no evidence of increased spasticity. No joint deformities, swelling, increased warmth, ligamentous laxity, or subluxations were noted in any of the extremities.

Diagnosis

Physical Therapist Practice Pattern 5H: Impaired Motor Function, Peripheral Nerve Integrity, and Sensory Integrity Associated with Nonprogressive Disorders of the Spinal Cord.

What types of problems might be suspected at this time?

The therapist reexamined the patient and concluded that the patient was experiencing complications related to poikilothermia. One neurologic complication with a spinal cord injury is the inability to regulate body temperature. With damage to the spinal cord, the hypothalamus may no longer control cutaneous blood flow or regulate sweating. The patient may lack the processes of vasoconstriction in response to cold and vasodilation in response to heat and lose the ability to shiver. The patient may also lack thermoregulatory sweating below the level of the lesion, which may inhibit the necessary evaporative cooling effects of perspiration in warm environments. To compensate, the patient may become diaphoretic and perspire above the segmental level of the spinal cord lesion. As a result of these thermoregulatory changes, the external environmental temperature profoundly affects the patient. The therapist noticed that the patient was always wearing thick, heavy-duty sweatpants and sweatshirts with a wool afghan wrapped around him whenever he was seated in his wheelchair. Furthermore, after performing a bedside session one afternoon when the patient stated he was not feeling well enough to receive therapy in the gym, the therapist noticed that the knob on the thermostat in the patient's room was turned all the way up to maximum heat.

Prognosis

The therapist anticipated that in approximately 1 week the patient would be able to fully participate in interventions.

GOAL

The patient and family will receive education on poikilothermia and demonstrate 100% compliance within 3 to 5 days, to regulate the patient's body temperature and facilitate increased participation in therapy sessions.

Intervention

After a spinal cord injury, the patient and his family face major lifestyle changes. The health care team provided accurate information as early as possible, and teaching about the effects of spinal cord injury was included in the therapy treatments. The patient and family were taught about autonomic dysfunction and the patient's inability to control body temperature. They were informed that his persistent low-grade fever and excessive sweating were the result of his excessive clothing and increased room temperature. They were instructed to rely heavily on the sensory input from the head and neck regions to assist in determining appropriate environmental temperatures. Because of the patient's and family's low educational levels, the therapist chose to use both verbal education and pictorial explanations to facilitate effective learning.

Outcome

After the patient and family were educated about poikilothermia, the patient's room temperature was adjusted appropriately, and his clothing consisted of sweat pants and a long-sleeved shirt. His fevers subsided, and he was able to actively participate in his therapy without complaints.

RECOMMENDED READINGS

Baxter K, Russo S: *Physical therapy management of spinal cord injury: accent on independence*, Woodrow Wilson Rehabilitation Center, 1994.

Ciccone C: *Pharmacology in rehabilitation* (ed 3), Philadelphia: FA Davis, 2001.

Ekman L: *Neuroscience: fundamentals for rehabilitation*, Philadelphia: WB Saunders, 1998.

Kingsley R: *Neuroscience*, Philadelphia: Lippincott Williams & Wilkins, 2000.

O'Sullivan S, Schmitz T: *Physical rehabilitation assessment and treatment* (ed 4), Philadelphia: FA Davis, 2001.

Watchie J: *Cardiopulmonary physical therapy*, Philadelphia: WB Saunders, 1995.

LEARNING OBJECTIVES

The reader will be able to:

1. Identify the effects on bowel and bladder control related to a conus medullaris spinal cord injury.
2. Describe a multidisciplinary approach necessary to successfully treat a patient diagnosed with a conus medullaris spinal cord injury.

The reader should know that a 30-year-old African-American male sustained a spinal cord injury from a motor vehicle accident after falling asleep at the wheel. The patient was found to have an L1 burst fracture with 80% collapse and retropulsion of fragments with resulting neurologic compromise. The patient underwent posterior stabilization with instrumentation and fusion, and 3 weeks later was transferred to a facility for rehabilitation with a conus medullaris spinal cord injury.

On physical therapy examination, the patient had an unremarkable past medical history without any abuse of drugs or alcohol, and he was functionally independent before his accident. The patient was to wear a TLSO clamshell brace when out of bed, in addition to bilateral compression stockings.

Physical therapy interventions focused on improving bed mobility, transfers, quality of gait, elevations, balance, and patient education. The patient was very motivated and achieved significant gains over the first 2 weeks of therapy. Despite this increased level of function, there was concern, for the patient became incontinent of bowel about every other day during physical therapy sessions. Not only was this frustrating and embarrassing to this young patient, but it also caused premature termination of the sessions, providing a barrier to the patient's further progress. In addition, the patient's insurance company noticed how well the patient was performing functionally and was pressuring for an early discharge. The discharge date was approaching quickly, and there was only a short time to maximize this patient's rehabilitation potential.

What would be the appropriate response in this situation?

Examination and Evaluation

HISTORY

The patient lived with his mother in a two-story home that had 13 steps with no railings. He worked at a factory where he performed heavy-lifting duties, and he understood that he would have to find a different occupation secondary to his injury. Medications included Rocephin as an antibacterial drug to prevent infection, Ambien for insomnia, Percocet as needed for pain, Colace as a stool softener, and Dulcolax suppository with digital stimulation to aid bowel evacuation.

SYSTEMS REVIEW

The patient was a very pleasant young male in no acute distress. He was alert and oriented to person, place, and time, and his cognition was intact. S1 and S2 heart sounds were noted, but no S3 or S4 sounds were appreciated. The lungs were clear in all fields bilaterally, and no rales, rhonchi, or wheezing were auscultated. The patient had a healing chest tube site in place postpneumothorax while acutely hospitalized, in addition to a stage II coccygeal pressure ulcer.

TESTS AND MEASURES

Manual muscle testing revealed 3+/5 strength bilaterally in ankle dorsiflexors and plantarflexors and 4–/5 strength in hip abductors, hip extensors, and knee flexors. All other areas exhibited grade 5/5 strength. During dermatome testing, the patient was unable to detect light touch in the L5-S1 segmental innervations. In addition, in accordance with the physician's evaluation, numbness was indicated in the perianal area and genitalia, with a vague bulbocavernosus reflex. In terms of functional status, the patient transferred wheelchair to and from bed with contact guard, performed all bed mobility with minimal assistance, and ascended and descended five stairs with one rail with contact guard. During gait assessment, the patient ambulated 150 feet on a level surface without an assistive device with contact guard. The therapist did not notice any difficulties with toe clearance, push-off, or knee control, but did appreciate "loose, swinging" hips bilaterally during lower extremity stance phases, characteristic of a Trendelenburg gait. Standing, dynamic, unsupported balance was fair.

Diagnosis

Physical Therapist Practice Pattern 5H: Impaired Motor Function, Peripheral Nerve Integrity, and Sensory Integrity Associated with Nonprogressive Disorders of the Spinal Cord.

Prognosis

Based on examination and evaluation data, the therapist estimated that a 2-week period would be necessary for the patient to fully participate in interventions.

How might physical therapy sessions become more efficient when the patient suffers from bowel incontinence on such a consistent basis?

The conus medullaris, anatomically located at the inferior border of the first lumbar vertebrae, is the terminal point of the spinal cord. After injury to the conus medullaris, autonomous (or nonreflex) neurogenic bowel and bladder develops, producing signs and symptoms similar to a lower motor neuron lesion. A lesion in this area damages the reflexive emptying circuit of S2-S4, producing flaccid, paralyzed musculature.

GOALS

1. (Nursing goal) The patient will decrease the number of bowel accidents by 100% within 1 to 2 weeks.
2. The patient will participate in physical therapy sessions 100% to facilitate increased functional mobility, within 1 to 2 weeks.

Intervention

The patient's lack of bowel control became a major issue due to its negative effects on the rehabilitative effort and the resulting emotional distress that the patient experienced. While the therapist spoke with the patient about the bowel program he was following while at the facility, the patient stated that the nursing staff arranged an every-other-day schedule that was performed in the evening. Furthermore, on inquiring about the patient's bowel schedule before his injury, the therapist learned that the patient had a bowel movement in the morning, every day. Considering the patient's previous bowel habits, the therapist discussed altering the patient's program with the nursing staff, suggesting that the bowel program be changed to the morning, every day, to acknowledge the patient's previous bowel habits.

Outcome

The nursing staff was agreeable to the therapist's request, and they helped the patient develop a bowel program that was consistent, timely, and regular. Once the patient was placed on a routine schedule where his bowel was "trained," he experienced therapy without any negative interruptions and became functionally independent before discharge.

RECOMMENDED READINGS

Baxter K, Russo S: *Physical therapy management of spinal cord injury: accent on independence*, Woodrow Wilson Rehabilitation Center, 1994.

Ciccone C: *Pharmacology in rehabilitation* (ed 3), Philadelphia: FA Davis, 2001.

Ekman L: *Neuroscience: Fundamentals for rehabilitation*, Philadelphia: WB Saunders, 1998.

Kingsley R: *Neuroscience*, Philadelphia: Lippincott Williams & Wilkins, 2000.

O'Sullivan S, Schmitz T: *Physical rehabilitation assessment and treatment* (ed 4), Philadelphia: FA Davis, 2001.

LEARNING OBJECTIVES

The reader will be able to:

1. Identify the functional skills that a spinal cord injury patient gains with the ability to roll.

2. List six techniques that may be used to facilitate rolling.

The reader should know that an 18-year-old, single, unemployed African-American male sustained a spinal cord injury from a high-speed motor vehicle accident 3 weeks earlier. Computed tomography scan revealed a fracture dislocation and subluxation of C6-C7. The surgical procedures involved fixation, fusion, and instrumentation. The patient also presented with an ORIF of his left olecranon fracture and scalp lacerations. The patient was transferred to a facility 3 weeks later with an examination consistent with C7-T1 ASIA level B quadriparesis (Table 16-1).

On physical therapy examination, the patient had an unremarkable medical history for hypertension, diabetes, or other chronic medical conditions. The patient had experienced two previous motor vehicle accidents, resulting in a pelvic fracture that was now healed. The patient denied any alcohol or drug abuse and was functionally independent before the latest accident. The patient was to wear an abdominal binder and Miami-J collar when out of bed, in addition to a left arm splint and bilateral pressure-relief ankle-foot orthoses (PRAFOs) and compression stockings.

During the initial physical therapy sessions, interventions focused on wheelchair mobility using a manual chair, transfers using a sliding board, sitting balance, bed mobility, increasing tolerance to vertical positioning using a tilt table, and patient education. The patient made moderate improvements in most aspects of physical therapy, but continued to experience difficulty with bed mobility, especially rolling supine to side-lying.

What would be the appropriate response to this patient's specific functional limitation?

TABLE 16-1
ASIA IMPAIRMENT SCALE

ASIA IMPAIRMENT SCALE
☐ **A** = **Complete:** No motor or sensory function is preserved in the sacral segments S4 to S5.
☐ **B** = **Incomplete:** Sensory but not motor function is preserved below the neurologic level and includes the sacral segments S4 to S5.
☐ **C** = **Incomplete:** Motor function is preserved below the neurologic level, and more than half of key muscles below the neurologic level have a muscle grade less than 3.
☐ **D** = **Incomplete:** Motor function is preserved below the neurologic level, and at least half of key muscles below the neurologic level have a muscle grade of 3 or more.
☐ **E** = **Normal:** motor and sensory functions are normal.

CLINICAL SYNDROMES
☐ Central cord
☐ Brown-Sequard
☐ Anterior cord
☐ Conus medullaris
☐ Cauda equina

From American Spinal Cord Injury Association: International Standards for Neurological and Functional Classification of Spinal Cord Injury, Chicago, 1996, p 26. Used with permission.

Examination and Evaluation

HISTORY

The patient lived with his parents and younger sister in a double-wide mobile home. He was WBAT on his left upper extremity and was in no acute distress. Medications included Lovenox as a deep vein thrombosis prophylaxis, Didronel as a prophylaxis to avoid heterotopic ossification, Senekot as a laxative, Dulcolax suppository with digital stimulation, and ibuprofen for pain relief.

SYSTEMS REVIEW

The patient was alert and oriented to person, place, and time, and cognition was within normal limits. No clubbing, cyanosis, or edema was noted, and dorsalis pedis pulsations were 2+ bilaterally. No evidence of joint deformities, increased warmth, ligamentous laxity, or subluxations in the trunk or extremities was seen. The lungs were clear on auscultation and percussion in all fields bilaterally. Stage I bilateral heel pressure ulcers, as well as healing scalp lacerations, were noted. Vital signs were temperature, 98.1° C; heart rate, 80 beats per minute (bpm); respiratory rate, 20 bpm; and blood pressure, 132/70 mm Hg in the supine position.

TESTS AND MEASURES

Motor strength was 5/5 grossly in bilateral upper extremities, 2/5 in trunk musculature, and 1/5 in bilateral hip movements. There was no presence of a motor component in the knees and ankles bilaterally, yet passive range of motion was within normal limits in the lower extremities. Sensation was intact to C7 bilaterally with the presence of "spotty" sensation below the level of injury. Sacral sparing was equivocal, as per physician evaluation, and proprioception was intact in the feet.

Diagnosis

Physical Therapist Practice Pattern 5H: Impaired Motor Function, Peripheral Nerve Integrity, and Sensory Integrity Associated with Nonprogressive Disorders of the Spinal Cord.

What recommendations helped facilitate rolling from supine to side-lying?

Rolling is a functionally significant skill that, once mastered, improves overall bed mobility, assists in dressing, and allows necessary positional changes to aid pressure relief and skin inspection. This skill helped this patient with a spinal cord injury develop functional patterns of movement by requiring him to use his upper extremities and trunk with momentum to move the lower extremities.

Prognosis

The therapist predicted that the patient would become independent in bed mobility within 2 to 3 weeks.

GOALS

1. The patient will demonstrate supine to right and left side-lying with the use of bilateral 1-pound wrist cuff weights, bilateral leg loops, and PNF upper extremity patterns with minimal assistance 100% of the time within 1 week.
2. The patient will demonstrate supine to right and left side-lying with only the use of PNF upper extremity patterns independently 100% of the time within 2 weeks.

Intervention

Various techniques can assist with supine to side-lying rolling, depending on the patient's functional level. For this patient, pillows were initially placed under one side of the pelvis and scapula to initiate rotation in the direction of the roll. One may also choose to provide manual assistance to these areas at the beginning of the roll when the maximum effects of gravity occur, and reduce assistance as the patient moves more easily. Because the patient's cervical orthosis restricted his neck movements, he relied on his upper extremities and trunk to complete the task. The patient was instructed to maintain extension in both arms, while symmetrically and rhythmically rocking his arms and head from side to side to create enough momentum to roll. Various upper extremity PNF patterns, such as D1F, reverse-chop, and lift patterns, were also used. Additional strategies to aid rolling included using wrist cuff weights to help increase momentum and using leg loops to position the lower extremities. The patient pulled up on the loops and crossed his ankles so that the upper limb was toward the direction of the roll. This positioning facilitated hip and lower extremity rotation as the upper extremities worked to complete the task. During the rolling movement, the patient coordinated a deep inspiration halfway through the roll, for once the shoulders were rotated, contraction of the diaphragm assisted with rolling.

Outcome

The patient's active-assisted movements gradually progressed to independent active supine to side-lying rolling. With the accomplishment of this task, the patient was educated on skin inspection of his sacrum with the use of a long-handled mirror. He also performed pres-

sure relief while in bed and further assisted his occupational therapist with lower extremity dressing. Furthermore, the physical therapist was able to initiate more advanced mat activities to help the patient become as functionally independent as possible.

RECOMMENDED READINGS

Baxter K, Russo S: *Physical therapy management of spinal cord injury: accent on independence*, Woodrow Wilson Rehabilitation Center, 1994.

Ciccone C: *Pharmacology in rehabilitation* (ed 3), Philadelphia: FA Davis, 2001.

O'Sullivan S, Schmitz T: *Physical rehabilitation assessment and treatment* (ed 4), Philadelphia: FA Davis, 2001.

O'Sullivan S, Schmitz T: *Physical rehabilitation laboratory manual*, Philadelphia: FA Davis, 1999.

LEARNING OBJECTIVES

The reader will be able to:

1. Summarize the challenges inherent in the management process of an adult with mental retardation who exhibits simultaneous and interactive impairments in neuromotor, musculoskeletal, developmental, cognitive, and affective domains.

2. Identify a functional management strategy that takes into consideration the interactive effects of common impairments associated with mental retardation.

3. Discuss the need, when working with a mentally retarded adult, for innovatively developing, modifying, and sharing with other providers a habilitation plan of care that promotes best function within the individual's environment.

4. Determine that an important outcome of the patient management process is the assurance that the habilitation plan of care is acceptable to the patient.

Examination

HISTORY

The patient was a 50-year-old male resident in a group home for adults with mental retardation. He had diagnoses of cerebellar atrophy, degenerative joint disease of the hips and knees, seizure disorder, and mental retardation. His medical history over the previous 6 months included numerous falls, with frequent lacerations to the head. Group home staff reported a fall frequency of one per week. He had been provided with one-to-one staffing/close monitoring at the group home, because most of his falls occurred at the group home. His seizure disorder was not completely controlled by medication. He had a generalized type seizure of 30 seconds duration approximately every other month. His most recent seizure medications were phenobarbital, dilantin, and neurontin. At the time of interview, the patient weighed 184 pounds, but his weight had been as high as 204. His "ideal weight" as listed in his medical chart is 125 pounds.

The patient attends a day program at another agency. He is required by the agency to use a wheelchair for mobility at all times.

He does not use a wheelchair at the group home. His yearly physical examination results state "restricted activity" and "needs to be well supervised with ambulation." He was referred for "physical therapy evaluation and treatment as needed" by his family practice physician.

The physical therapy–related goals of the group home staff were for the patient to be able to get up from the floor safely, decrease his number of falls, and keep him ambulating.

SYSTEMS REVIEW

Cognitive status. The patient demonstrates perseverative behavior. He prefers to side sit or heel sit on the floor and engage in either shredding paper or sorting small objects for extended periods. He avoids eye contact when he does not feel comfortable with individuals. When angry, he hits the floor repeatedly with his hand. When angry, he also has thrown himself backward from a standing position, resulting in personal injury. He does not attempt to engage people but rather prefers to do activities by himself. He effectively communicates a strong sense of what activities he will and will not allow others to engage him in within the group home. Staff reported that he can say a few words, indicate no by shaking his head, and respond to simple commands.

Neurologic status. The patient can stand independently and cross his midline with his hand, but the action is tenuous. He can reach down and touch the floor to pick up items with and without using one hand for support. For control of balance, he uses an ankle strategy; the use of knee and hip strategies for balance was not noted. He prefers manual support from staff or a support surface when walking short distances within the group home.

Strength. The patient can rise to standing from a half-kneeling position but required a support surface for balance. A complete determination of functional strength was not possible, because the patient was not willing to perform a full range of functional activities for this evaluation.

Joint range of motion. The patient demonstrated no significant joint contractures. A gross screen of upper extremity joint range of motion revealed a range within normal limits. He did not appear to have any pain associated with the degenerative joint disease of his hips and knees. His heel cords were mildly tight, as evidenced by approximately 10 degrees of active dorsiflexion bilaterally.

Posture and ambulation skills. The patient stood with a wide base of support. He had a markedly forward head posture with forward rounded shoulders, forward flexed trunk, and a pendulous abdomen. He walked with a varying step length. Staff reported that the quality of his ambulation skills tended to degenerate as the day progressed.

Diagnosis

Physical Therapy Practice Pattern 5A: Primary Prevention/Risk Reduction for Loss of Balance and Falling.

Prognosis

GOAL

The patient will reduce the risk of falling through therapeutic exercise, balance training, and lifestyle modification.

The expected range and number of visits per episode of care is between three and five.

EXPECTED OUTCOMES

Within 3 months, the patient will:

1. Demonstrate the ability to reach down without external support and pick up an item from the floor three times within 2 minutes without loss of balance.
2. Walk about the group home without seeking the use of a supporting surface (table, countertop).
3. Decrease the reported number of falls per week by 100%.
4. Demonstrate 75% compliance with the plan of care.

DISCHARGE PLAN

The patient will be discharged from physical therapy services when there is a consensus among the group home manager and staff that the patient is capable of safely walking about the group home with an assistive device and without a contact guard or the need to remain within staff's field of vision.

Intervention

The patient completed the Tinetti balance and gait assessment to quantify his walking and balance skills with and without a cane. His risk for fall without the cane, and whether using the cane objectively decreased his risk for fall, were assessed.

A dietetic consult was initiated to develop an appropriate weight control plan. Weight reduction will reduce stress on his hip and knee joints and move the patient's center of gravity more within his base of support.

An attempt was made to get the patient to use a weighted pistol-grip cane through a specific training program. The weighted cane bottom might make it easier for him to place the cane on the floor with each series of steps. It might also make him less likely to use the cane as an offensive weapon should he have a behavioral outburst while ambulating.

The patient was observed walking about the group home in his bare feet to assess whether this provides better somatosensory feedback from his feet and helps improve his balance skills. Using a protective helmet or headgear was considered. The appropriateness of the patient's footwear was evaluated, and footwear that can help enhance static and dynamic balance was recommended.

Outcome

The patient completed the Tinetti balance and gait assessment without using a cane to quantify his ambulation and balance skills and his risk for falls. His scores were 5/12 for the gait portion, 2/16 for the balance portion, and 7/28 for the combined gait/balance score. A score below 19 is considered to represent a high risk for falls. With a total score of 7/28, this patient is considered to be at significant risk for falls. The Tinetti assessment tool was not attempted with the patient using a cane, because he was unable to use the cane appropriately.

An attempt was made to have the patient use a tip-weighted, pistol-grip cane to provide him with a wider base of support. He walked with the weighted cane in his hand, but did so with the cane never coming in contact with the floor despite frequent verbal and physical cues from the therapist. After three trials of ambulation training with the cane, the patient walked with the therapist to his bedroom door. He opened the door, threw the cane against the far wall, closed the door, and then walked away from the therapist. A rolling walker was also tried, but the patient did not like how it impeded his independent walking and simply pushed it enough to move it off to the side so he could walk around it.

The patient's two pairs of sneakers were assessed to determine whether his footwear was assisting or impeding his balance while standing and walking. With his flexed, forward rounded posture, his sneakers (which had angled, full soles) tipped him forward and displaced his center of gravity forward on his base of support. Flat, full-soled sneakers, which did not elevate his heels and alter his center of gravity within his base of support, were determined to be the most appropriate footwear to aid balance. The group home staff was told that the patient did not need to wear his sneakers when home. It was hoped that walking without the sneakers at home might give the patient enhanced proprioceptive input, thereby enhancing his balance and possibly preventing some falls.

The use of an assistive walking device was not feasible with the patient, because he did not want to use one even though it was believed that he would benefit from its use. An alternative recommendation was made for the patient to walk with the assistance of staff when at all possible. Staff would simply offer an arm as an external support.

Discussion was initiated with the group home supervisor as to whether the use of a protective helmet was reasonable and feasible for the patient. The patient has a strong aversion to any type of headgear, and is even unwilling to wear a baseball cap or a stocking cap. Therefore, the use of any protective headgear was considered unfeasible.

Group home staff followed up with the dietetic consultation and recommendations regarding the optimum footwear for the patient. The issue of walking about the group home in bare feet was pursued but evaluated by the group home supervisor versus the physical therapist.

In consultation with the group home staff and the referring physician, and considering that the anticipated goal and outcomes were not achieved, this episode of physical therapy care was discontinued.

Discussion

Discontinuing the plan of care was deemed appropriate for the following reasons:
1. The plan of care was not acceptable to the patient. The balance difficulties and risk for falls were not considered problems by the patient, and were of concern only to those working with him. The patient had no perceived need to be actively engaged in a program of therapeutic exercise

related to addressing loss of balance and risk of falling. Therefore, the gait training with an assistive device was discontinued.

2. This was a situation wherein a patient with mental retardation refuses physical therapy services that would be in his best interest. This is a confrontation between two opposing moral principles, patient autonomy and therapist beneficence. It would be in the patient's best interest to comply with the plan of care (therapist beneficence), yet he very clearly indicates, in his own way, that the plan of care is not acceptable to him (patient autonomy). It is not appropriate to choose an action deemed to be beneficial for a patient simply because a caregiver thinks he or she knows better. That would be paternalism. The patient's right to make choices for his life and to express those choices must be acknowledged. This patient had made it clear what his choices were regarding the issues of loss of balance and risk of falling. There was no other appropriate course but to implement his free decision.

RECOMMENDED READINGS

Bertoli DB: Mental retardation: focus on Down syndrome. In Tecklin JS (ed): *Pediatric physical therapy* (ed 3), Philadelphia: Lippincott Williams & Wilkins, 1999.

Long T, Toscano KH: Older persons with developmental disabilities. In Guccione AA (ed): *Geriatric physical therapy* (ed 2), St Louis: Mosby, 2000.

Davis CM: Identifying and resolving moral dilemmas. In *Patient practitioner: an experimental model for developing the art of healthcare* (ed 3), Thorofare, NJ: Slack, 1998.

Davis CM: Influences of values on patient care: foundation for decision making. In O'Sullivan SB, Schmitz TJ (eds): *Physical rehabilitation: assessment and treatment* (ed 4), Philadelphia: FA Davis, 2001.

LEARNING OBJECTIVES

The reader will be able to:

1. Differentially diagnose lumbopelvic instability, and other causes of low back pain, that can be associated with urinary urge incontinence, especially in a female.

2. Explain the relationships between the pelvis, pelvic floor, low back pain, and urinary incontinence.

3. Discuss the importance of evidence-based practice (EBP) in physical therapy as it relates to women's health.

4. Make sound clinical decisions based on EBP, thorough history, systems review, appropriate tests and measures, and diagnosis.

5. Develop a prognosis and an appropriate plan of care for a patient with a complex presentation of low back pain, pelvic pain, and urinary urge incontinence.

Examination

HISTORY

General demographics. The patient was a 42-year-old, left-hand-dominant, Caucasian female. Her obstetrician referred her to physical therapy via telephone, with a diagnosis of incontinence and low back pain. Her primary language was English, and she had a bachelor's degree in business administration. She was employed as the administrative assistant to the CEO of a cellular telephone manufacturing company.

Social history. The patient was married with two children, a 3-year-old girl and a 6-month-old boy. Her husband traveled 3 or 4 days every week, but was usually home on the weekends.

Functional status and activity level. The patient's hobbies included reading and singing, and she was an avid runner. She had completed five marathons in the past 6 years, and before the last pregnancy ran at least 5 days a week, for a cumulative distance of up to 60 miles per week. She stopped running as soon as she found out she was pregnant, because she did not want to take any chances of a second miscarriage. She started again 3 months after the delivery, to help her lose her "baby weight." Her job involved prolonged episodes of sitting, spending at least 6 hours a day at the computer. She had not been able to work for the past week because of severe back and leg pain. She was not able to drive a car, and had a friend drive her to therapy. Before this current episode of low back pain, she had been independent with all activities of daily living (ADL) and had had no problem fulfilling her roles of mother, wife, and employee. At the time of her first visit she could not pick up her baby or her daughter because of the pain, and had to rely heavily on help from others (i.e., mother, friends) with household chores as well as care of her family.

General health status. The patient had always been in excellent health and she felt great until a week ago. At the time of the first visit, she reported trouble sleeping at night, because she couldn't get comfortable, leading to a feeling of exhaustion. She worried about what was going on, and if she would ever be the same again.

Social/health habits. The patient is a nonsmoker and a social drinker (up to two drinks of wine or beer, no more than 5 nights a week).

Family history. The patient's father had arthritis of the neck, hips, and low back. Her mother died at age 61 of myocardial infarction. She had no other significant family history.

Medications. The patient currently takes Advil and Aleve. During previous episodes of low back pain she took only Advil, which always proved effective. She took no other prescription medications.

Medical/surgical history. *Cardiovascular:* History of borderline high blood pressure for about 1 year, up until 2 years ago. Since she started transcendental meditation, she stopped taking medication and no longer has high blood pressure.

Endocrine: De Quervain's thyroiditis 6 years ago, with no residual effects.

Gastrointestinal: A perforated colon and a temporary ileostomy 8 years ago. The cause of the perforation was unknown.

Genitourinary: Frequent urinary accidents starting about 3 years ago and worsening since her last pregnancy. Her main problem is that she sometimes cannot make it to the bathroom in time. She also has nocturia three or four times a night and a history of four bladder infections in the past 10 years, but none within the past 2 years. She takes Cranactin (an over-the-counter herbal substitute) daily for urinary tract health. She reports no pain or burning with urination and no problems with bowel movement.

Gynecologic/obstetric: Gravida (pregnancies) 3, para (delivered) 2, miscarriage 2 years ago. Her first pregnancy was without complications. Her daughter was born at 39 weeks, via vaginal delivery in a semireclining position, using natural childbirth, without epidural anesthesia. Her second pregnancy ended in a miscarriage at 10 weeks. During her last pregnancy, she gained 52 pounds. She had a vaginal delivery in a semireclining position, after about 10 hours of labor. She had an episiotomy and a tear through slightly more than half of the perineal body. The tear was sutured but has remained tender. Since the delivery, sexual intercourse has been painful, and she cannot use tampons because of the pain on insertion.

Integumentary: Unremarkable.

Psychological: Unremarkable, except for anxiety related to the pain and how it affects her daily life.

Pulmonary: Unremarkable.

Prior hospitalizations and preexisting medical conditions: Emergency abdominal surgery in 1996 with a temporary ileostomy, and a reversal 4 months later. Appendectomy at age 6. Otherwise unremarkable.

Musculoskeletal: Hyperextension injury to the low back at age 18. History of occasional back pain, described as a nagging feeling in the small of her back with prolonged sitting or standing and with "window shopping." That pain is always significantly less when she exercises regularly, including doing sit-ups. Two right-ankle sprains more than 10 years ago.

Neuromuscular: Unremarkable.

Other clinical tests. Radiography or magnetic resonance imaging was not done. No specific urinary tests were performed. The gynecologist believed that the symptoms of incontinence were related to her pregnancy and would improve over time. When the patient called the gynecologist about the back pain, she was referred to physical therapy without an examination.

Current condition/chief complaint. The patient expressed concern about how her back pain interfered with her home, work, and social life. She was not currently receiving any therapy, other than the Aleve and Advil. This was the first time she had had this much back pain. Current symptoms were severe pain in the small of her back, on the right. This pain radiated into the right hip and buttock, and somewhat down the right leg. Occasionally, when putting weight on the right leg, the pain shot down the right leg, and at those times was sharp and stabbing. The pain was also present with moving from sitting to standing and vice versa. She had had some back discomfort over the past 3 months, because of the extended long hours spent sitting at work. Seven days before her first physical therapy visit, she had come home from a 5-mile run, and when she bent over to pick up her 6-month-old son, something "snapped." The instant pain brought her to her knees. The pain had gotten somewhat better since then. Sleeping was a challenge, because she could not find a comfortable position in bed.

Goals and expectations: The patient wants to eliminate the pain, so she can participate in her daily life activities. She also desires relief of the pelvic pain and her incontinence to normalize those aspects of her life as well.

SYSTEMS REVIEW

Cardiovascular/pulmonary. Blood pressure, 128/78 mm Hg with the patient sitting, taken on the right arm; heart rate, 82 beats per minute (bpm), taken at the radial pulse on the right arm; respiratory rate, 13 bpm; no apparent presence of edema of the extremities.

Integumentary. No apparent skin breakdown or discolorations were noted on the trunk and extremities.

Musculoskeletal. *Gross symmetry:* When sitting, weight bearing was greater on the left side; forward head tilt and rounded shoulders were also noted. No other deficits clearly apparent.

Gross range of motion (ROM): With the patient sitting, ROM of neck and upper and lower extremities was within age-appropriate norms. ROM for forward flexion of the lumbar spine was painful and limited to 50% for all movements. The hip exhibited limited right internal rotation (by approximately 25%) and limited bilateral adduction (by approximately 25%); neither was described as painful, but both were described as "tightness" by the patient.

Gross strength: Results of myotome testing were strong and symmetric throughout, except for the right L5 myotome (right great toe extension).

Neuromuscular. Gross sitting balance appeared normal. The patient's gait as she walked into the clinic was antalgic, with decreased weight bearing on the right side, slow deliberate movements, and lack of reciprocal arm swing and trunk rotation, requiring support on her mother's arm. Transfer stand to sit was very slow and deliberate and clearly painful, with guarding of back movement (in an apparent attempt to avoid trunk rotation and flexion as much as possible) and decreased weight bearing on the right side.

Communication/cognition. The patient exhibited no apparent deficits, other than distress over the pain, and her inability to function in her normal roles in society. She answered all questions appropriately and was able to understand and follow complex commands.

Based on the information from the history and systems screen, what tests and measures were appropriate and why?

The patient's main complaint was pain, pointing to the need for a thorough pain assessment. Because of the weakness of the L5 myotome and the complaint of radiating pain, sensory testing of the dermatomes was done to rule out potential spinal involvement. The apparent asymmetry of posture could be due to a muscular imbalance, misalignment in the spine or the sacroiliac joint (SIJ), or lumbopelvic instability.[1] Therefore, muscle length and strength testing and assessment of joint accessory mobility of the spine, the SIJ, and the pubic symphysis were indicated. Palpation was needed to further pinpoint the possible source of the low back pain and also to check whether the low back and the radiating pain could be reproduced, which can help identify the structures involved.

Because of the patient's antalgic gait, a thorough gait analysis and balance assessment were performed to identify possible contributing factors.

According to the *Gynecological Manual* from the American Physical Therapy Association's Section on Women's Health,[2] it is very important that a vaginal evaluation of the pelvic floor be performed to obtain specific information about tone, location/presence of pain and tenderness, sensation, function, and strength of the pelvic floor muscles and other supporting structures. This evaluation was performed.

Another key assessment step was to have the patient keep a bladder diary to provide more specific information about fluid intake (amount and type) and output. Ideally, this should be a 2-week diary.

What could have been causing the patient's complaints?

Because of the patient's history of occasional low back pain, particularly during episodes of decreased exercise and hyperextension injury, as well as her recent pregnancy and the hormonal changes associated with that, lumbopelvic instability[1] was considered a very likely cause of the complaints.

The urinary complaints appeared to be a result of urge incontinence and were more than likely based on learned behavior, although the pregnancy and the delivery trauma certainly could have aggravated the symptoms. The pelvic floor pain was probably related to the episiotomy and subsequent tearing and suturing of the perineal body. Research indicates that the more severe tears are most likely to occur after an episiotomy, and that suturing of the scars results in greater and more prolonged complaints.[3,4]

TESTS AND MEASURES

Based on the aforementioned considerations, an evidence-based practice (EBP) search on the evaluation of lumbopelvic instability,[1–3] and the American Physical Therapy Association's *Gynecologic Manual and Guide to Practice*,[5] the following tests and measures were performed:

- *Bladder diary for 1 week*, for inclusion in treatment planning.
- *Gait, locomotion, and balance*, as described in *Systems Review*. Ambulation while performing dual tasks (counting backward by seven and carrying a filled water glass) reduced speed of ambulation by 50% on a 3-meter long, level surface. Walking speed was 1.0 meters/second. No backward ambulation was tested because of pain and the patient's discomfort with the request. Static balance in standing was within norms. Perturbations were not tested because of the patient's pain on standing and guarding of movement.
- *Integument of the perineum*. The patient's pelvic floor was examined with patient in hook lying, draped. A 1-inch-long scar was visible at 12 o'clock. The first half-inch,

closest to the vagina, was straight, whereas the more posterior half-inch was more ragged looking. The entire scar looked red and swollen and was tender to the touch, rated at 5/10. Adhesion was present intermittently over the entire length of the scar, for at least 75% of the total scar. No other deficits were noted.

- *Joint integrity and mobility*, including joint accessory mobility of SIJ and special tests for SIJ mobility. No decreased mobility of the lumbar spine was apparent. Hypomobility was noted on the right SIJ.
- *Motor function of the pelvic floor.* No apparent coordination difficulty with contraction of the pelvic floor was noted. Co-contraction of abdominal and gluteal muscles, as well as the adductors, was noted with pelvic floor contraction. There was minimal lifting of the pelvic floor with contraction.
- *Performance of muscles* of the abdomen, back, and pelvic floor, including observation, palpation, strength, and biofeedback. Strength of the upper abdominals measured 4/5; that of the lower abdominals, 2+/5. The patient was unable to stabilize her lower back when asked to perform activities with either lower extremity while supine. Muscle spasm was noted on palpation of lumbar paraspinal musculature and quadratus lumborum bilaterally, but greater on the right side than on the left side. Palpation of the right SIJ was tender on the lateral aspect and reproduced some of the back pain. A trigger point was located in the right piriformis muscle. On the pelvic floor, the tear adhered intermittently throughout the episiotomy scar, and was tender to palpation. Increased tone was noted, as was an inability to fully lower the pelvic floor to a normal resting position. The baseline reading on surface electromyelography was 3.5 mV; the maximum reading with contraction was 6 mV. Clock palpation elicited tenderness externally at 12, over the scar, and on the right at 3. Vaginal tenderness was noted at 12, and a trigger point was found in the right obturator internus. The strength of the pelvic

floor muscles was evaluated as 2+/5. The patient was able to hold for 6 seconds, became fatigued after three repetitions, and could do five fast 1-second contractions before she fatigued. Strength of right great toe extension was 3/5.

- *Pain.* The patient described the pain as 10/10 when present as a shooting pain down the leg during weight bearing and otherwise as 6/10 at rest, increasing to 8/10 with prolonged sitting, standing, or walking and on transfers. The patient characterized the pain as a grabbing pain in the low back on the right, radiating into the right buttock and somewhat to the back and outside of the right upper thigh.
- *Posture in walking, standing and sitting.* Walking posture exhibited forward head position, rounded shoulders, and increased lumbar lordosis. Decreased hip extension was noted on the right side during terminal stance. Standing posture was marked by a forward head position, rounded shoulders, increased weight bearing on left, bilateral genu recurvatum, pronated feet (left greater than right), slight lateral shift to the left of the spine on the pelvis, right iliac crest lower than left; forward rotation of right ilium (right PSIS higher, right ASIS lower); increased external rotation of the right foot. The sitting position was marked by a forward head position, rounded shoulders, and weight bearing mostly on the left side.
- *ROM of hip.* Extension: right, 5 degrees; left, 8 degrees. Flexion: 130 degrees bilaterally. Internal rotation: left, 45 degrees; right, 30 degrees. External rotation: 45 degrees bilaterally. Abduction: 20 degrees bilaterally. Thomas test: positive on the right side.
- *Reflex integrity* (particularly to rule out neurologic causes of urinary and back pain problems). Patellar reflexes: 2+/4 (normal). Achilles tendon: 2+/4. Anal sphincter reflex: present and symmetrical. Cough reflex: pelvic floor reflexive contraction present. No sign of urine leakage with cough.
- *Sensory integrity.* The patient correctly identified pain sensation and light touch

5/5 in bilateral lower extremities, except for lateral aspect of right foot (correctly identified 2/5). Sensation of the perineum was 5/5 for light touch. The patient refused pain assessment of perineum.

PROBLEM LIST

- Radiating back pain
- Decreased ROM of lumbar spine
- Muscle-guarding in low-back musculature
- Pelvic floor scar adhesion and pain
- Pelvic floor increased tone, inability to fully relax
- Pelvic floor weakness
- Frequency of urination and leaking of urine a minimum of seven times a week.
- Trigger point in right obturator internus and right piriformis
- Abdominal muscle weakness
- Piriformis and hip flexor tightness
- Postural deviation, patient unaware of proper posture and body mechanics
- Antalgic gait
- Decreased SIJ mobility on right; forward rotation of right ilium
- Inability to perform functions as wife, mother, and employee
- Unable to drive a car; dysfunctional with transfers; disrupted sleeping pattern

Diagnosis

Physical Therapist Practice Pattern 4D: Impaired Joint Mobility, Motor Function, Muscle Performance, and Range of Motion Associated with Connective Tissue Dysfunction.

Prognosis

Over the course of 3 months of therapy, with visits initially three times per week for 1 week, decreasing to two times per week for 2 weeks, and further decreasing to once every other week or less, the patient will return to her preinjury level of daily work, home, community, and leisure activities with minimal to no pain. ROM, muscle performance, muscle tone, joint mobility, and posture will all return to age-normal ranges.

GOALS

Within 6 weeks, the patient will:

1. Decrease back pain to 2/10.
2. Return to work, life, and social activities, with pain no higher than 4/10.
3. Be able to do home ADLs and IADLs with normal body mechanics and pain no greater than 4/10.
4. Report decreased pelvic floor pain to 3/10.
5. Exhibit decreased pelvic floor resting activity to 3 mV.
6. Decrease adhesions to 50% of the episiotomy scar from 75%.
7. Exhibit decreased trigger point tenderness in piriformis and obturator musculature, to 4/10.
8. Demonstrate increased pelvic floor strength, from 2+/5 to 3/5.
9. Exhibit increased strength of the lower abdominals, to 3/5, increasing lumbopelvic stability.
10. Correctly answer all questions about posture, bladder training, and bladder irritants.
11. Have normal muscle strength of piriformis, adductors, and hip flexors, as demonstrated by normal ROM for hip motion.
12. Decrease the number of urinary accidents from seven per week to three per week.
13. Increase the voiding interval to 1 hour.

The following goals were anticipated to be reached in 2 to 3 months, with visits no more than bimonthly during the last 2 months of care. The patient will:

1. Function independently in all work, life, and social activities, with back pain no greater than 2/10.
2. Increase the voiding interval to 3 hours.
3. Demonstrate independence with all exercises.
4. Report decreased pelvic pain, to 0–1/10.
5. Report no pain on intercourse or tampon insertion.
6. Demonstrate absence of scar adhesion.
7. Demonstrate a resting tone of the pelvic floor 1.5 to 2 mV.
8. Exhibit pelvic floor strength of 3+/5 or greater.

9. Reduce the number of urinary accidents to fewer than one per week.
10. Demonstrate independence with the home exercise program and decision making on progression of exercises.

DISCHARGE PLAN

demonstrated the ability to function independently with subjective reported pain levels below 2/10 during all social, home, and work ADLs, and when the number of urinary accidents had decreased to less than one per week, and when the patient and therapist believed that the patient could perform her home exercise program independently, including progression of intensity and frequency of exercises.

Additional recommendations include referral back to the obstetrician or a urologist for urinary testing to rule out other pathologies, including unstable detrusor muscle and obstruction to urine flow, and to evaluate bladder and kidney function.

Intervention

Ultrasound (US) is frequently used to promote wound healing and soften scar tissue. Based on the results of an EBP search, the benefits of US for postpartum perineal pain and dyspareunia are neither conclusive nor definite.[6] Because there seems to be a small improvement of perineal pain from using US compared with placebo, intermittent US was used over the perineum, using a water-filled condom for the first three treatments only, for 5 minutes per treatment.

The systematic review on guidelines for treatment of low back pain by the Philadelphia panel showed that the only intervention that significantly improved low back pain and function for acute low back pain was return to normal activities.[7] The intervention for the back pain was decided to include grade 2 joint mobilization to the right SIJ and the use of muscle energy techniques to derotate the right ilium. Trigger point massage of the piriformis trigger point was also performed, as was myofascial release of the pelvis and the abdominal region. Based on the findings of the Philadelphia panel, no other interventions were performed, other than patient education on proper posture for standing, sitting, and walking and proper body mechanics at both home and work. The patient was also educated about the optimal workstation setup at work, and on energy-preservation techniques while performing work-, home-, and community-related activities.

Other specific interventions were performed as follows:

- Soft tissue: Scar massage, along with myofascial release of pelvic girdle, lumbar spine, and pelvic floor, as well as the scar adhesions, were performed. Trigger point massage was also performed vaginally to the obturator internus.
- Strengthening: Pelvic floor strengthening exercises (starting with two sets of 5-second hold contractions, with a 5-second rest in between, followed by 10 quick [1-second] contractions) twice a day while supine; lower abdominal muscle strengthening exercises,[8] and lumbar stabilization exercises.
- Biofeedback: To reduce the tone of pelvic floor and teach isolation of the pelvic floor contraction.
- Patient education: Topics include fluid intake, type of fluid, behavior modification to normalize voiding pattern, self-massage of perineal body, body mechanics for lifting of children, sitting posture at work, desk setup, and postural training.
- Stretching of tight hip flexors, piriformis, and abductors.

Outcome

It took the patient 2 weeks to complete her urinary diary. On the last day of the second week, she reported no incidence of urine leakage, and the voiding intervals had increased from a maximum of 45 minutes to 75 minutes. The maximum void volume had increased from 3 oz to 4 oz. She still had to get up three times per night to void.

After the third visit (she was seen three times a week that first week), the adhesions had reduced to about 50% of the scar. US was discontinued at that time, but scar massage and myofascial release continued. The perineal pain had decreased, and tampon insertion was no longer painful, although sexual intercourse remained painful. The radiating pain in the leg was centralizing. The PSIS and ASIS were symmetrical and pain free. The patient was able to walk at a rate of 2 meters/second, and the pain in the back and leg with functional activities had decreased to 5/10. Pelvic floor tone remained high, and no measurable increase in the strength of muscle contractions was seen.

The frequency of treatment was decreased to twice a week for 1 week, and then to once a week for the next 3 weeks. After 2 weeks of treatment, the patient was able to return to work, with pain levels not exceeding 4/10 throughout the day. Pain was present only in the low back area, and was no longer continuous. The perineal scar was without adhesions at this point, and piriformis and obturator trigger points were no longer present. Scar massage and trigger point massage were discontinued. Stretching and strengthening exercises were continued, and the strength of the lower abdominals increased to 3/5, to aid reduction of lumbopelvic instability. Hip ROM also improved.

Subsequently, the frequency of treatment was further reduced to once every other week for 2 weeks, and then to once a month, as the patient demonstrated the ability to perform all her exercises independently, perform scar massage correctly, and progress her exercises appropriately. Treatment at this time consisted mostly of biofeedback with pelvic floor muscle training. Resting tone reading was now consistently at 2 mV, and her peak contraction was at 8 mV. Urine leakage incidents had decreased to between one and two per week, and voiding intervals had increased to 2½ hours, with normal fluid intake. Sexual intercourse was no longer painful.

After a total of 12 visits, the patient was discharged, having met all of her goals.

Discussion

The patient's motivation to resume running, as well as her other social, work, and home activities, and her adherence to her home exercise program resulted in an excellent outcome, despite the complexity of the case. The support from her mother and friends made it possible for her to take the time during the day to do her exercises.

Based on EBP studies on the use of pelvic floor muscle training for the treatment of urinary incontinence of women, this was added to the behavior modification training of her urge incontinence.[9] EBP has shown some (albeit not conclusive or definite) evidence that adding pelvic floor muscle training to behavioral training is more beneficial than either pelvic floor muscle training or behavioral alone in the treatment of urge incontinence.[11]

Because the pelvic floor is attached to the pelvis, any adhesions and changes in tone can create distortion of the pelvis. Therefore, it was important to treat the pelvic floor, as well as strengthen the lumbopelvic stabilizing muscles, to prevent recurrence of the pelvic torsion. Restoring the muscle balance of the pelvis, low back, and hip was also important to maintain proper alignment.

REFERENCES

1. http://www.coca.com.au/newsletter/2001/sep0101a.htm.
2. Wilder E (ed): *The gynecological manual*, Alexandria, VA: American Physical Therapy Association, Section on Women's Health, 2000.
3. http://www.changesurfer.com/Hlth/episiotomy.html.
4. http://www.gentlebirth.org/format/woolley.html.
5. American Physical Therapy Association: Guide to physical therapist practice, second edition, *Phys Ther* 81:1, 2001.
6. Hay-Smith EJ: Therapeutic ultrasound for postpartum perineal pain and dyspareunia, *Cochrane Database Syst Rev* 2002:CD000495.
7. Philadelphia Panel: Evidence-based clinical practice guidelines on selected rehabilitation interventions for low back pain, *Phys Ther* 81:1641, 2001.
8. Hodges PW: Is there a role for transversus abdominis in lumbopelvic stability? *Man Ther* 4:74, 1999.
9. Hay-Smith EJ, Berghmans LC, Hendriks HJ, et al: Pelvic floor muscle training for urinary incontinence in women, *Cochrane Database Syst Rev* 2001:CD001407.

LEARNING OBJECTIVES

The reader will be able to:

1. Identify the specific signs that aid in differentially diagnosing potential musculoskeletal disorders that can affect the hip region.
2. Identify a treatment strategy that a patient may comply with and that is appropriate for the patient's injury and lifestyle.
3. Identify common special tests for the hip joint, including the Thomas test and the Faber test.

Examination

HISTORY

The patient was a 38-year-old athletic male who presented with a main complaint of right intermittent inner groin and thigh pain commencing 3 weeks earlier, after he began jogging in preparation for a 35-and-over basketball league. His symptoms increased in severity, frequency, and duration. He received no treatment before his first visit except for resting from playing basketball over the past weekend. He worked out regularly using free weights and a stationary bicycle, and he occasionally used the swimming pool. He stated that he did not stretch with any regularity. His job was mainly sedentary.

The patient reported that stepping up stairs immediately increased his pain from 3/10 to 7/10. This pain settled within 3 minutes. He also stated that jogging immediately increased his pain to 8/10; however, this eased within 5 to 10 minutes. Lying supine with his hip slightly flexed and a pillow under his thigh eased the pain to 0/10 after approximately 20 minutes. His hip was stiff on waking, and the symptoms were variable with activity during the day. He noticed that he awakened when turning in bed most nights.

The patient walked into the clinic with a mildly antalgic gait and a decreased stride length on the right. He reported a "clicking" in his right hip. His general health was good, with no recent unexplained weight loss. The only medication he was taking was ibuprofen; however, he suffered from exercise-induced asthma and used an oral inhaler as needed. No radiographs had been taken of the painful hip.

SYSTEMS REVIEW

Integumentary system. There was noticeable bruising in the region of the right groin as well as the right upper thigh region. At the time of assessment, the bruising was green-yellow and, according to the patient, had decreased considerably.

Gross symmetry. No significant differences in symmetry were seen. Leg length and weight bearing were deemed equal.

Palpation. There was marked tenderness on palpation of the origin of the adductor and pectineus muscles. Palpation reproduced the patient's complaint. There was also some spasm located in the deep paravertebral muscles from L2-L5 on the right.

Joint range of motion. Active hip flexion was 120 degrees with a stiff capsular painful end feel. Extension was –10 degrees (active) and also stiff and painful. Active hip abduction was 15 degrees with a painful, soft capsular end feel. External rotation was measured actively as 35 degrees, and a stiff capsular end feel was once again noted. All other ranges were normal and pain free.

Strength. Muscle strength in all groups was full and pain free except for adduction and flexion, which were 4-5/5 and inhibited by pain.

Special tests. Straight leg raise was limited to 80 degrees on both sides. A positive Thomas test was noted for the right hip flexors, with a 10-degree hip flexion contracture. The Faber test was also positive for the reproduction of pain on the right.

Other joints. The lumbar spine was limited by 20% during forward flexion and side flexion to the right. There was an associated increase in pain at the end of the available range. ROM from posteroanterior central vertebral pressures at L3-L4 were limited by 25% and caused an increase in low-back and thigh pain. The knee had a full range of pain-free motion.

This patient could have presented with a lumbar spine disorder with associated referred pain into the groin and hip region or presented with a simple hip joint pathology. Which signs suggested hip joint pathology?

The following signs suggested hip joint pathology:
• Decreased ROM
• Decreased muscle power at the hip joint
• Pain inhibiting motion and muscle strength
• Positive signs elicited by special tests

The patient was diagnosed with a second-degree groin strain of the right adductor muscles.

Diagnosis

Physical Therapist Practice Pattern 4E: Impaired Joint Mobility, Motor Function, Muscle Performance and Range of Motion Associated with Localized Inflammation.

Prognosis

It was anticipated that the patient would return to his sport within 3 to 4 weeks of following an appropriate treatment protocol. The expected number of visits was between four and six, spread over 4 weeks.

SHORT-TERM GOALS
The patient will be able to:
1. Walk and ascend stairs without pain within 2 weeks.
2. Be independent in a home stretching routine after two treatment sessions.

3. Demonstrate independent use of heat/ice for a home program by the second treatment session.
4. Sleep without waking from pain within 2 weeks.

LONG-TERM GOALS
The patient will:
1. Have full pain-free ROM by the end of the fourth week.
2. Be able to jog without pain by the end of the sixth week.
3. Be independent with a home strengthening program and sport specific drills for basketball by the end of the sixth week.

Intervention

Initial treatment consisted of deep transverse friction to the affected muscle origins. Pulsed ultrasound was applied to the affected muscle origins to break down any cross-bridges that had developed in the scar tissue deposited since the time of injury. The patient was given ice massage to decrease any soreness from treatment and to limit any fresh inflammatory response triggered by the friction massage. A stretching protocol was put in place, and the patient was given a home exercise program consisting of stretching and icing activities to be carried out two to three times per day.

Once ROM was regained, stretching exercises were commenced, with only straight-line motion used. As time progressed and the patient's pain decreased, ROM increased, and strength increased, more functional activities were implemented and sport-specific drills undertaken.

Outcome

The frictions were applied for approximately 60 seconds initially, and any reaction was recorded. Because no adverse effects were seen, friction massage was then applied for 10 minutes. The pulsed ultrasound treatment afforded some initial pain relief and localized treatment to the site of injury. Because of the delay in seeing this patient, pulsed ultrasound was applied on the first day of treatment and used throughout. Pulsed ultrasound was also used to assist in realignment of the fibers of any scar tissue that had been deposited.

The ice massage decreased the soreness produced by the stretching and deep transverse friction massage. This was also incorporated as part of the home exercise program. Passive stretching of the damaged muscle tissue aided realignment of the scar tissue deposited during the repair process. The extensibility of the muscle tissue needed to be increased before the patient could return to activity. Strengthening exercises were withheld for the first week to decrease pain and attempt to regain the lost ROM. Regaining ROM must be accompanied by appropriate strengthening within the newly regained range. Before discharge, the patient had to demonstrate specific drills and exercises required for a return to his previous level of activity.

Reexamination

On reexamination after 2 weeks, it was found that stepping up stairs caused an immediate increase in pain, which settled after just 1 minute and registered as only 4/10 on the pain scale. Jogging still caused an immediate increase in pain, which settled after only 3 minutes and registered as 4/10. The patient's hip was still slightly stiff on waking; however, it no longer awakened him when he turned in bed.

The patient's antalgic gait had resolved, and his ROM had improved to near-normal levels. The lumbar spine signs decreased considerably, with only a mild increase in symptoms occurring at the end of the range. Some slight tenderness persisted in the adductor and pectineus muscles; however, there was no longer any spasm associated with the deep paravertebral muscles between L2 and L5 on the right. The Thomas test was reassessed at 10 degrees of hip flexion contracture on the right, and the Faber test was still positive for reproduction of pain on the right hip.

Having considered the initial treatment and the long-term goals set, what would be an appropriate course of treatment that would continue the positive progress achieved thus far?

An appropriate course of treatment would be to continue with deep transverse friction to treat the localized injury, and review the home exercise program and ensure that the patient was not overdoing it. It was found that the patient had been attempting to push his home exercise program too quickly, and he was advised of the potential risks involved with this course of action. A new home exercise program was devised that included a number of safe sport-specific activities to give the patient the feeling that he was returning to his chosen sport, but in a controlled way.

DISCHARGE

Discharge from physical therapy occurred when the patient had regained full active pain-free ROM in all directions and could perform specific exercise tests without developing pain or stiffness.

RECOMMENDED READINGS

Starkey C, Ryan J: *Evaluation of orthopedic and athletic injuries*, Philadelphia: FA Davis, 1996.

Norris CM: *Sports injuries: diagnosis and management* (ed 2), Oxford, UK: Butterworth-Heinnemann, 1998.

Zuluaga M, Briggs C, Carlisle J, et al (eds): *Sports physiotherapy: applied science and practice*, Melbourne, Australia: Churchill Livingstone, 1995.

American Physical Therapy Association: Guide to physical therapist practice, second edition, *Phys Ther* 81:1, 2001.

LEARNING OBJECTIVES

The reader will be able to:

1. Discuss the pathomechanics associated with pylon fractures.
2. Identify and differentiate clinical signs and symptoms associated with compartment syndrome.
3. Identify and discuss potential sources of error in managing patients with pylon fractures that may lead to complications.
4. Identify appropriate referral sources for patients.
5. Describe how to apply controlled forces using manual techniques, positioning, and aquatic therapy to facilitate healing.

Background on Diagnosis

Pylon fractures are usually associated with a high-impact injury in which the calcaneus and talus are driven up like a wedge through the tibia and fibula, splitting the interosseus membrane and fracturing the tibia and fibula

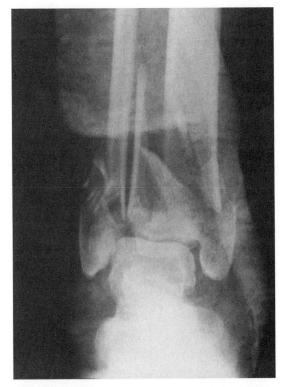

FIGURE 20-1 A pylon fracture. (From Daffner RH: *Clinical radiology: the essentials,* ed 2, Lippincott Williams and Wilkins, Baltimore, 1993.)

(Figure 20-1). Common complications associated with this type of injury include loss of limb length, abnormal function of the talocrural and subtalar joints, compartment syndrome, and neurovascular changes. Arthrosis or other complications occur in about 50% of patients with this type of fracture; approximately 26% of affected patients will require ankle-joint fusion.[1,2]

The reader should know that a 39-year-old postal worker sustained a pylon fracture of the right lower extremity while on vacation when he fell off an 8-foot-high wall and landed on the right leg. The patient underwent an open reduction to remove bony fragments. An external fixator was applied to maintain traction through the fracture site in an attempt to restore and maintain limb length during healing. He was initially prescribed Keflex (for infection), Demerol (for pain), and coumadin (as an anticoagulant).

The surgeon recommended a short-term stay of 3 weeks in the hospital rehabilitation unit to ensure compliance with postoperative restrictions. The insurance company approved a 3-day stay with follow-up home care nursing and one or two home visits by physical therapy. The orthopedic surgeon was concerned about the stability of the fracture and recommended the patient remain non–weight-bearing for a minimum of 5 weeks and that he not perform any active muscle contraction or range of motion (ROM) exercises for the first 3 weeks.

The patient developed an infection 3 weeks after surgery and was readmitted to the local hospital for a 3-day course of intravenous antibiotics and surgical debridement of the infection. Radiographs at the time revealed initial healing of the fractures but with several areas of malunion. The ankle joint space appeared to be maintained at this time. The physician extended the restrictions of no ROM and no weight bearing for an additional 4 weeks.

The external fixator was removed at 12 weeks, and the patient was placed in a removable walking cast brace, but remained non–weight-bearing. The patient was eventually referred for outpatient physical therapy 14 weeks after the initial surgery. The prescription read: "begin PROM of the ankle, gait training @ 10% of body weight through involved LE, AAROM for DF and PF only for the first 3 weeks, and general full body strength and conditioning program. Avoid excessive traction or compression through the involved extremity!"

What clinical signs and symptoms would lead the examiner to believe a compartment syndrome may have been developing?

Examination

HISTORY

The patient was a 39-year-old male, married with three children ages 3, 6, and 10 years. He was employed full time as a mail carrier and walked 5 to 8 miles per day on his route, which he described as moderately hilly. His mail route had more than 500 stops. He was a member of the Postal Workers Union; the Union did not offer light duty for his position. He supplemented his income by officiating high school football and track one to three times per week. His wife had a high school education and had been staying at home with their youngest son. Since the initial home visit the patient had gained 15 pounds. He was ambulating non–weight-bearing on the involved extremity and used axillary crutches, but admitted he had not been walking more than 200 feet at a time since the injury and had for the most part avoided stairs.

He reported pain at 6/10 (0, no pain; 10, worst pain) in the involved lower extremity when it was in a dependent position for more than 10 minutes. He described the pain as a general ache or pressure. He expressed concern over the strange sensations that he had been feeling in the involved leg and described them as itching, burning, cold, or hot, but he was not able to associate any of the feelings with any particular activities or positions. There was significant atrophy throughout the involved lower extremity. All incisions appeared to be well healed, with no drainage present.

Blue to reddish-purple mottling was noted with the involved extremity in a dependent position. When moved to a supported position, the extremity returned to a healthy pink color within a few minutes.

The patient was taking Advil or Alleve for the pain, which reportedly provided some relief. The patient stated he was anxious to progress with weight bearing so that he could return to work. His employer could hold his current position as a mail carrier for only 2 months. The patient's and family's understanding of the patient's severity of injury and the need to adhere to restrictions appeared to be a concern.

SYSTEMS REVIEW

The results of a systems review were unremarkable.

TESTS AND MEASURES

ROM and strength of the uninvolved extremities were within normal limits as described in standard texts.[2-5] The involved extremity was slightly limited for knee flexion, with 110/115 degrees, and extension, with –5/0 degrees active/passive (A/P) range of motion. Ankle motion A/P was limited to 5 degrees of plantarflexion from neutral. There was no dorsiflexion past neutral and no measurable inversion or eversion. Vital signs[3,4,7] were stable. Circulation[3-5,7] was impaired in the involved extremity in dependent positions, with lower extremity swelling and mottling within 10 minutes of placement in a dependent position. The patient also complained of paresthesias with the onset of swelling and discoloration. Sensation[3-5,7] was intact for the uninvolved extremity but inconsistent for the involved extremity in dependent versus elevated positions with light touch. Gait with crutches was independent on level surfaces for short distances, less than 200 feet, secondary to reported paresthesias in the lower leg. The patient required contact guard on stairs with crutches because of difficulty coordinating movements at the time of the initial examination.[3-5] The patient was independent in performance of activities of daily living and IADLs.[3,4]

Evaluation

PROBLEMS (FUNCTIONAL LIMITATIONS AND IMPAIRMENTS)

1. The patient was the sole provider for his family. He was not able to return to work until fully recovered. Given the type and severity of his injury, he would be out of work between 4 and 8 months.[3,4]
2. Decreased activity level. The patient had not been active since the initial injury, which had resulted in decreased cardiovascular endurance, weight gain, and muscle atrophy.[3,4]
3. Potential for limited return of ROM and strength in the involved extremity.[1,2]
4. Motivation. The patient was anxious to return to work, which would help with compliance with the exercise program; however, he did not fully understand the need to allow proper healing to occur.[3]
5. Neurovascular signs and symptoms. The patient needed to be monitored closely to avoid development of complications commonly associated with pylon fractures.[1-3,5,6]

Diagnosis

Physical Therapist Practice Pattern 4I: Impaired Joint Mobility, Motor Function, Muscle Performance, and Range of Motion Associated with Bony or Soft Tissue Surgery.

Compartment syndrome was ruled out because of the reduction of symptoms with change of position.

Prognosis (including plan of care)

Over the course of 1 to 8 months, the patient will demonstrate optimal joint mobility, motor function, muscle performance, and ROM and the highest level of functioning in home, work (job/school/play), community, and leisure environments. The expected number of visits was between 6 and 70.[3,4]

PHYSICAL THERAPY PLAN OF CARE

The long-term goals (2 months) of physical therapy were to prevent complications and restore maximal function in the involved extremity. Short-term goals (1 to 2 weeks) included patient and family education and facilitation of healing through symptom management and initiation of therapeutic interventions using controlled forces.

Based on the initial examination findings, what type of activities and positions were most beneficial for exercise?

Might this patient have benefited from any other services?

Intervention

Aquatic therapy was used initially to allow the patient to work on gait training, stretching and AAROM.[3,4,7,8] The principals of buoyancy were used to limit weight bearing (deeper water for less weight bearing) and to facilitate ROM in the hip, knee, and ankle by changing the position of the extremity in the water.

A portion of each session was spent on patient and family education related to healing, and the need to adhere to weight-bearing limitations and proper performance of exercises.[3,4]

Manual techniques as described by Kisner and Colby[9] and O'Sullivan and Schmitz[3] were used to facilitate (P/A/AA) ROM and stretching for the involved extremity. Exercises were initiated in an elevated position to aid venous return. By the fourth week of treatment, the patient gained control of the muscles in the involved extremity. The time to onset of paresthesias, edema, and discoloration in the involved extremity when in dependent positions increased so the exercise positions were progressed to more-dependent positions.

Cardiovascular activities included the use of an upper-body ergometer initially. The patient was also able to swim using only arm strokes at first, progressing to straight leg kicking and eventually to whip kicks. He was progressed to a stationary bike at approximately 4 weeks as ROM improved and weight bearing increased. After 8 weeks of treatment, the patient received clearance to begin ambulation on a treadmill.[3,4,7,8]

The patient was referred to other health care providers, including a social worker, psychiatrist, and vocational counselor.

Outcome

At the time this case was reported, the patient was 7 months postinjury and was still receiving physical therapy. He was ambulating with a cane for distances up to 1.5 miles. He still had significant limitations in ankle ROM and fluctuating edema in the lower leg and foot. He had not yet returned to work but had entered a job-retraining program.

REFERENCES

1. Netter FH: *The Ciba collection of medical illustrations, vol 8, musculoskeletal system. Part III: trauma, evaluation, and management,* Summit, NJ: Ciba-Geigy, 1993.
2. Placzek JD, Boyce DA: *Orthopedic physical therapy secrets,* Philadelphia: Hanley & Belfus, 2001.
3. O'Sullivan SB, Schmitz TJ: *Physical rehabilitation assessment and treatment* (ed 4), Philadelphia: FA Davis, 2001.
4. American Physical Therapy Association: Guide to physical therapist practice, second edition, *Phys Ther* 81:9, 2001.
5. Evans RC: *Instant access to orthopedic physical assessment,* St Louis: Mosby, 2002.
6. Goodman CC, Snyder TE: *Differential diagnosis in physical therapy* (ed 3), Philadelphia: WB Saunders, 2000.
7. Bates A, Hanson N: *Aquatic exercise therapy,* Philadelphia: WB Saunders, 1996.
8. Ruoti RG, Morris DM, Cole AJ: *Aquatic rehabilitation,* Philadelphia: Lippincott, 1997.
9. Kisner C, Colby LA: *Therapeutic exercise foundations and techniques* (ed 3), Philadelphia: FA Davis, 1996.

Case **21**

LEARNING OBJECTIVES

The reader will be able to:

1. Assess information from the interview of a patient with paresthesias in the upper extremity and identify the most pertinent information.

2. Identify which aspects of a postural examination and upper quarter screen are likely to provide the most pertinent information when performing a physical examination.

3. Decide which special tests may be most helpful in making an accurate diagnosis.

4. Decide which intervention may be most appropriate for this patient.

Examination and Evaluation

HISTORY

The patient was a 37-year-old female with a diagnosis of right carpal tunnel syndrome. She reported pain and intermittent paresthesias in her right hand that developed over the past three months. She also reported difficulty using her hand to perform household chores as well as in her job in a factory. She stated that her hand easily tired and she often dropped objects. The pain and paresthesias were described as being primarily in the thumb and the second and third fingers. She stated that the pain and paresthesias originally began after she used a new piece of equipment at work that required her to frequently turn knobs that she found difficult to turn. The patient continued to work. She requested to be transferred to a different piece of equipment at work, but her request was denied.

The patient reported a past medical history of a motor vehicle accident 2 years earlier in which she injured her neck. She was seen by a physical therapist three times per week for 2 months. She reported still having some residual stiffness in her neck, especially in the mornings. Further, she noted having similar symptoms in both hands during her last pregnancy 4 years earlier. Those symptoms lasted for several months after the pregnancy and then slowly dissipated. (Carpal tunnel syndrome is common during preg-

nancy.[1]) She reported no other significant past medical history.

The patient wore a neutral wrist splint for the past 2 weeks at work as directed by her physician. The purpose of the splint was to reduce stress in the carpal tunnel.[2] (The carpal tunnel is least restricted in the neutral position. Wrist extension of approximately 20 degrees, as is commonly seen in a resting or cock-up splint, could produce tension on the median nerve in the carpal tunnel.) The patient reported that wearing the splint for the last 2 weeks did not change her symptoms.

The patient was prescribed Naproxen, 250 mg t.i.d., but stopped taking the drug after only 6 days because of stomach irritation. She reported smoking half a pack of cigarettes per day and denied any use of alcohol or recreational drugs. The patient was a single parent living in an apartment with two children ages 7 and 15 years. She worked in a factory that produced plumbing fixtures.

What parts of the interview were most significant in determining the course of the physical examination?

The pattern of paresthesias appeared to be most closely associated with a median nerve distribution. Other possible sources of paresthesias in the hand, such as injury to nerve roots or other peripheral nerves or diabetic neuropathy, must be ruled out.[3,4] Determination of the source of paresthesias should be clarified with sensory testing. Because of the patient's past medical history associated with the motor vehicle accident, cervical spine involvement must be ruled out. If the median nerve was involved, it must be determined where that involvement has occurred.

What areas should be examined concerning the type of work that the patient performed?

Further questions concerning the new piece of equipment revealed that the patient used this piece of equipment most of the day. The equipment required her to often turn a knob, with her right hand, in a counterclockwise direction, against resistance. She also complained of pain and fatigue in her forearm and hand and paresthesias in her hand by the end of the day.

PHYSICAL EXAMINATION

The patient was 5 feet 8 inches tall and weighed 140 pounds. She presented in standing with a mild forward head position and mild thoracic kyphosis. An upper-quarter screen[5] revealed that cervical range of motion was mildly limited in extension and rotation bilaterally. There was no complaint of symptoms with either motion or pressure. All upper extremity motions were within normal limits (WNL), with no complaint of symptoms with motion or overpressure. All resisted isometrics in the upper extremities were found to be strong and painless. A dermatome scan was normal in all regions of the upper extremities, except that the patient reported decreased sensation on the palmar side of the first, second, and third fingers of the right hand. Deep tendon reflexes were found to be normal and symmetrical for the biceps (C5), brachioradialis (C6), and triceps (C7) muscles.

What was determined from the findings of the upper-quarter screen?

The results of the upper-quarter screen appeared to rule out the cervical spine as a source of her symptoms. No symptoms were reproduced with cervical motion or pressure to the cervical spine. The sensory changes identified did not appear to be in a particular nerve root pattern, such as C6 or C7, because there was no loss of sensation in the forearm. The sensory pattern appeared to be that of the median nerve.

What other tests were required to clarify the extent of median nerve involvement and where?

The dermatome scan was not specific enough to enable detection of the involvement of muscles innervated by the median nerve, muscles innervated by other nerves, or the location of involvement. Careful sensory testing and manual muscle testing was therefore required.

More careful testing of the sensory pattern confirmed involvement of the median nerve. The patient was found to have paresthesias in the palmar surface of the first, second, and third fingers and the radial half of the fourth finger, as well as on the dorsal surface of the distal ends of the same fingers. Sensation was normal in the rest of the hand and in the forearm. Sensory loss resulting from diabetic or alcoholic neuropathy would tend to be in more of a "glove" pattern, involving all the fingers of the hand, and generally not in a specific nerve pattern.[3]

The amount of sensory loss can be clinically measured using a static two-point discrimination test, a moving two-point discrimination test, the Semmes-Weinstein monofilament test, or vibratory sensation testing.[4] The Semmes-Weinstein monofilament test was used for this patient. Test results revealed that the patient's sensory loss was moderate in nature (she was able to detect the sensation from a 2.83 monofilament) and confined to the regions of the hand innervated by the median nerve.

Sensory testing confirmed median nerve involvement. The median nerve was determined to be intact, however, because the patient had some sensation in that nerve distribution.

How could it have best been determined where the median nerve was involved?

Motor function of the median nerve was assessed to determine the location of median nerve involvement. Manual muscle testing revealed that all muscles innervated by the ulnar and radial nerves were 5/5. Results of MMT of muscles innervated by the median nerve were determined to be as follows:

- Pronator teres, 5/5
- Flexor carpi radialis, 5/5
- Flexor digitorum superficialis, 5/5
- Flexor digitorum profundus (to second and third fingers), –3/5
- Flexor pollicis longus, –3/5
- Abductor pollicis brevis, –3/5
- Flexor pollicis brevis, –3/5

Manual muscle tests determined that the median nerve was involved, but not all muscles innervated by the median nerve sustained involvement. It was determined that muscles innervated by the median nerve distal to the carpal tunnel were involved, as were several muscles innervated by the median nerve proximal to the wrist. This finding helped rule out the carpal tunnel as the primary source of the patient's symptoms. Both the sensory loss to the lateral three fingers and muscle weakness would explain why the patient reported dropping objects and having difficulty performing tasks at home and work.

What special tests could have been performed to more clearly identify the source of the patient's problem?

Upper limb tension tests were performed. The test using the median nerve bias reproduced the patient's symptoms.[6] Tinel's sign[7] at the wrist and at the upper palmar forearm was positive. (To elicit Tinel's sign, the examiner taps along a nerve trunk; a positive Tinel's sign involves reproduction of paresthesias within the sensory distribution of the nerve in question. Tinel's sign can be positive distal to any point along which the nerve has been affected.)

What was the potential value of isometric testing in ascertaining the source of the patient's problem?

Resisted isometric testing of the forearm reproduced the patient's symptoms with repeated resisted pronation but not repeated supination. The median nerve passes into the forearm between the two heads of the pronator teres.[8] Repeated resisted pronation may result in hypertrophy of the pronator teres and compression of the median nerve between the two heads of that muscle. The pronator teres, flexor carpi radialis, and flexor digitorum superficialis are all innervated by the median nerve proximal to the nerve traveling between the two heads of the pronator. The flexor digitorum profundus to the second and third fingers and the flexor pollicis longus are innervated distal to the median nerve passing between the two heads of the pronator, as are the muscles of the hand innervated by the median nerve (abductor pollicis brevis, flexor pollicis brevis, opponens pollicis, and first and second lumbricales).

The sensory pattern would be the same whether the nerve was compressed between the two heads of the pronator or in the carpal tunnel. The weakness in the hand muscles innervated by the median nerve would also be the same whether the nerve was compressed between the two heads of the pronator or in the carpal tunnel. The main difference considered in determining whether the median nerve was being compressed in the carpal tunnel or between the two heads of the pronator was the weakness found in the flexor pollicis longus and flexor digitorum profundus to the second and third fingers.[9] The upper limb tension test confirmed that the median nerve was involved, but the Phalen's and reverse Phalen's tests confirmed that the median nerve was not primarily affected at the wrist.

The physical therapy diagnosis was confirmed with an electromyogram (EMG) and nerve conduction velocity (NCV) test. The EMG determined that all muscles in the hand innervated by the median nerve were affected, whereas the muscles innervated by the ulnar nerve were not affected. The flexor digitorum profundus to the second and third fingers and the flexor pollicis longus were affected, and all other muscles in the forearm were normal. The NCV test showed slowing along the medial nerve from a point beginning just distal to the elbow.

What was a logical course of intervention for this patient?

Diagnosis

Physical Therapy Practice Pattern 5F: Impaired Peripheral Nerve Integrity and Muscle Performance Associated with Peripheral Nerve Injury.

Prognosis

GOALS

1. The patient will demonstrate control of small objects with her right hand without dropping them, so that she can perform dressing and household tasks, within 3 weeks.
2. The patient will display 5/5 muscle strength in all muscles innervated by the median nerve, so that she can perform all work tasks, within 4 weeks.

Intervention

A key strategy to ensure a successful intervention was to arrange for the patient to rest her right upper extremity from resisted pronation. Frequent resisted pronation caused hypertrophy of the pronator teres, resulting in compression of the median nerve as it passed between the two heads of the muscle. Ice and pulsed ultrasound over the pronator teres region was used to decrease inflammation. The patient also benefited from gentle stretching of the pronator teres and mobilization of the median nerve.[10] A gentle gliding of the median nerve freed up motion of the median nerve, enhancing the nerve's ability to glide between the two heads of the pronator

teres muscle. Care was taken not to stretch the nerve too aggressively. Symptoms should not be exacerbated during treatment. Excessive tension could further damage the nerve, resulting in further disability to the patient.

The patient was instructed to ice her anterior forearm at home after work and gently stretch into elbow extension, supination, and wrist flexion to glide the median nerve. She was instructed not to cause any reoccurrence of paresthesias while doing her exercises because this was a sign that she was stretching too aggressively and possibly irritating the nerve.

Outcome

Finally, the patient was permitted to switch to a different piece of equipment that did not require her to perform resisted pronation. As a result, she was able to continue working. On her breaks, she applied ice to her forearm just below the elbow three times per day. She was also seen in a local outpatient physical therapy clinic three times per week for 3 weeks. The patient made a full recovery, which included a return of normal sensation and strength of the right upper extremity.

REFERENCES

1. Jacobs JL: Hand and wrist. In Richardson JK, Iglarsh ZA (eds): *Clinical orthopedic physical therapy*, Philadelphia: WB Saunders, 1994.
2. Coppard BM, Lohman H: *Introduction to splinting: a clinical-reasoning and problem-solving approach* (ed 2), Philadelphia: Mosby, 2001.
3. Emanuele NV, Emanuele MA: Diabetic neuropathy: therapies for peripheral and autonomic symptoms, *Geriatrics* 52:40, 1997.
4. Tan AM: Sensibility testing. In Stanley BG, Tribuzi SM: *Concepts in hand rehabilitation*, Philadelphia: FA Davis, 1992.
5. Hertling D, Kessler RM: The cervical-upper limb scan examination. In Hertling D, Kessler RM (eds): *Management of common musculoskeletal disorders* (ed 3), Philadelphia: Lippincott, 1996.

6. Kleinrensink GJ, Syoeckart R, Mulder PG, et al: Upper limb tension tests as tools in the diagnosis of nerve and plexus lesions: anatomical and biomechanical aspects, *Clin Biomech* 15:9, 2000.

7. Magee DJ: *Orthopedic physical assessment* (ed 3), Philadelphia: WB Saunders, 1997.

8. Rosse C, Gaddum-Rosse P: *Hollenshead's textbook of anatomy*, Philadelphia: Lippincott-Raven, 1997.

9. Gerstner DL, Omer GE: Peripheral entrapment neuropathies in the upper extremity. Part 1: Key differential findings, median nerve neuropathies, *J Musculoskel Med* 3:14, 1988.

10. Elvy RL: Treatment of arm pain associated with abnormal brachial plexus tension, *Aust J Physiother* 32:225, 1986.

LEARNING OBJECTIVES

The reader will be able to:

1. Assess the information from the interview of a patient with anterior thigh and medial knee pain and identify the most pertinent information.

2. Identify which aspects of a postural examination and lower quarter screen are likely to give the most pertinent information when performing a physical examination.

3. Decide which special tests may be most helpful in making an accurate diagnosis.

4. Decide which intervention may be most appropriate for this patient.

Examination

HISTORY

The patient was a 59-year-old male who had a primary complaint of right anterior thigh and medial knee pain. He reported that the pain had increased gradually over the past 3 months and had become significantly worse within the past 2 weeks. He stated that the pain was most severe in the morning and gradually dissipated throughout the day. He had difficulty falling asleep because the right thigh and knee pain, and occasionally low back discomfort would wake him at night. He was employed as a heavy-equipment operator on a construction site.

The patient reported injuring his low back on the job on several occasions in the past. The most recent injury occurred 5 years earlier. Immediately after each injury, he was referred to physical therapy. Past physical therapy treatment included moist heat, ultrasound, massage, and therapeutic exercise. The patient was again referred to physical therapy by the company physician, with a diagnosis of quadriceps strain, and was given a prescription for naproxen. The patient reported engaging in recreational bowling two evenings per week, and stated that the pain was worse when he finished bowling. The patient indicated that he was 6 feet 4 inches tall and weighed 275 pounds.

What were the key findings from the interview?

Pain that is worse in the morning and relieved with activity can be a sign of osteoarthritis. Difficulty with sleep and pain waking a patient at night can indicate pain of nonmusculoskeletal origin.[1] Night pain is much less of a concern as long as the patient's symptoms can be explained with findings on physical examination. The history of past low back pain was significant for a possible source of his present symptoms. Pain in the anterior thigh may stem from pathology in the anterior thigh, lumbar spine, or knee or may be referred from the hip area.[1] Physical examination should address each of these possibilities.

With all of those possible sources of the patient's symptoms, where was the best place to begin the examination?

The examination began with a postural assessment and a lower quarter screen. This type of examination helped to rule out sources of the patient's symptoms.[2]

PHYSICAL EXAMINATION

The lower screen examination[2] revealed that the patient was limited in all directions of lumbar mobility (flexion, extension, side-bending right and left, and rotation right and left). He complained of stiffness in the low back with each of the motions but reported that none of the motions reproduced his right lower extremity pain. The motions were repeated with overpressure applied at the end range. Overpressure did not reproduce the symptoms in the thigh or knee. Multiple repetitions of each motion were then performed, also with no reproduction of symptoms. A dermatome scan was negative.

Resistive isometric examination[2] revealed that all muscle groups, including the quadriceps, were strong and pain free. Manual muscle testing of the quadriceps revealed a strength score of 5/5. Neither palpation of the quadriceps muscle or tendon reproduced any pain.

The patient was unable to do a squat without pain and tended to lean toward the left. Hip abductors on the right were found to be 4/5. Hip adductor, extensor, and flexor strength was found to be 5/5. Screening of lower extremity range of motion revealed limited mobility actively and passively in right hip flexion, abduction, internal rotation, and extension. All other lower extremity motions, including those of the right knee, were within normal limits and pain free. The right hip joint was limited in a capsular pattern[3] (flexion, abduction, internal rotation, extension) with a capsular end feel.[4] These two findings were indicative of a tight hip joint capsule.

What was concluded from the results of the examination thus far?

The lumbar screen appeared to rule out the lumbar spine as a source of the patient's symptoms.[2] A finding of strong and pain free, with resisted isometric testing of the quadriceps, was an indication that the muscle, tendon, or where the tendon attaches to the bone was not involved in the pathology.[2] The patient's inability to do a squat may be indicative of decreased mobility, pain, weakness, or a balance deficit in the lower extremities.[2]

When presented with these findings, what other special tests were then most appropriate?

Based on the patient's symptoms, Faber's test was performed. This test involves positioning

the patient supine with the knee flexed and the foot on the opposite tibia, then passively flexing, abducting, and externally rotating the hip. The test leg falling to the level of the opposite leg indicates a negative test.[5] The test revealed that the right leg was 4 to 5 inches higher than the left leg. The patient complained of pain with overpressure of the movement. Restricted motion, as indicated by the Faber test, may be indicative of tightness of the hip adductors, flexors, or hip joint capsule.

A scouring test was performed. This test involved flexing and extending, as well as abducting and adducting, the patient's hip while applying a compression force.[5] The patient complained of pain, and the examiner felt irregular movement at the hip joint, indicating possible degenerative changes of the joint surface.

A gait analysis was performed. The patient ambulated with a lateral lurch to the right. He also ambulated with a slightly flexed posture at the right hip. A lateral lurch may be a sign of either hip abductor weakness or a response to hip pain.[3] Manual muscle tests of the hip abductors produced a score of 5/5.

Further examination of the knee revealed that it was not tender to palpation and that range of motion was within normal limits. All ligamentous stability tests were normal and pain free, and meniscal tests were normal. These findings appeared to rule out the knee as a possible source of the patient's symptoms.

What were the results of the clinical examination?

The clinical examination appeared to show that the hip joint was the cause of the patient's symptoms. The hip joint is known often to refer pain to the anterior thigh and medial knee.[5] The patient's overall size and work history, as well as his history of operating heavy equipment, may have been a contributing factor to the development of hip osteoarthritis.[6]

What was a logical course of intervention?

Diagnosis

Physical Therapist Practice Pattern 4D: Impaired Joint Mobility, Motor Function, Muscle Performance, and Range of Motion Associated with Connective Tissue Dysfunction.

Prognosis

GOALS

1. The patient will be able to put on his shoes without pain in 2 weeks.
2. The patient will be able to ambulate 1000 feet without pain or gait deviation (lateral lurch) in 4 weeks.
3. The patient will be able to bowl without pain in 6 weeks.

Intervention

The patient's physical therapy program began with riding a stationary bicycle to warm the hip joint capsule and surrounding musculature.[7] After riding the exercise bicycle, the patient was manually stretched by the therapist into hip flexion, extension, abduction, and adduction to loosen the tight musculature surrounding the hip joint.[7] The hip joint was then mobilized, using joint capsule distraction techniques in an attempt to stretch the joint capsule.[7] The patient was given a cane to use in the left hand to decrease the compressive forces at the right hip joint.[3] The patient was instructed in a program of therapeutic exercise designed to maintain the increased range of motion and strength.[8] He was treated initially three times per week for 4 weeks, then two times per week for 2 weeks, and finally one time per week for 2 weeks. On discharge, he was instructed to continue with his home program permanently. He was able to discontinue the use of the cane and return to work after the first 4 weeks of therapy.

The strengthening exercises were begun slowly, with minimal resistance. Resistance was gradually increased over time. Endurance training was implemented to help the patient better tolerate a full day at work. Endurance exercises included stationary bicycle riding, free weights, and an offsite swimming program.

Outcome

The patient reported a gradual decrease in his pain. His gait improved until the lateral lurch was no longer evident. He was then able to discontinue the use of the cane. He was educated about the importance of maintaining good strength and flexibility of his hip. He was informed that maintaining proper strength and mobility could help to slow the progression of arthritis in his hip and help him avoid total hip replacement surgery.[9]

REFERENCES

1. Goodman CC, Snyder TEK: *Differential diagnosis in physical therapy* (ed 3), Philadelphia: WB Saunders, 2000.
2. Hertling D, Kessler RM: The lumbosacral-lower limb scan examination. In Hertling D, Kessler RM (eds): *Management of common musculoskeletal disorders* (ed 3), Philadelphia: Lippincott, 1996.
3. Barr AE, Backus SI: Biomechanics of gait. In Nordin M, Frankel VH (eds): *Basic biomechanics of the musculoskeletal system*, Philadelphia: Lippincott Williams & Wilkins, 2001.
4. Cyriax J: *Textbook of orthopaedic medicine. Volume I: Diagnosis of soft tissue lesions* (ed 7), London: Bailliere Tindall, 1979.
5. Magee DJ: *Orthopedic physical assessment* (ed 3), Philadelphia: WB Saunders, 1997.
6. McKinnis LN: Fundamentals of radiology for physical therapists. In Richardson KJ, Iglarsh ZA: *Clinical orthopedic physical therapy*, Philadelphia: WB Saunders, 1994.
7. Kisner C, Colby LA: *Therapeutic exercise: foundations and techniques*, Philadelphia: FA Davis, 2002.
8. Van Baar ME, Assendelft WJ, Dekker J: Effectiveness of exercise therapy in patients with osteoarthritis of the hip and knee, *Arthritis Rheum* 42:1361, 1999.
9. Salter RB: *Textbook of disorders of the musculoskeletal system* (ed 3), Baltimore: Williams & Wilkins, 1999.

LEARNING OBJECTIVES

The reader will be able to:

1. Assess the information from the interview of a patient with low back pain and lower extremity paresthesias and identify the most pertinent information.

2. Identify which aspects of a radiological examination may be most helpful to a physical therapist in determining accurate diagnosis.

3. Identify which aspects of a postural examination and lower-quarter screen are likely to give the most pertinent information when performing a physical examination.

4. Decide which special tests may be most helpful in making an accurate diagnosis.

5. Decide which intervention may be most appropriate for this patient.

Examination

HISTORY

The patient was a 62-year-old male with a diagnosis of lumbar strain. He reported that 2 weeks earlier, after a week of fly-fishing in Montana, he began experiencing pain in his low back and intermittent pain and paresthesias in the right lower extremity to the foot. The patient reported that the pain was worse with prolonged standing and prolonged walking but was relieved with sitting and lying in a fetal position. He denied any feeling of weakness in the lower extremities or any bowel or bladder changes.

The patient reported having past bouts of low back pain in his thirties and forties but no significant bouts for at least 15 years. He had often felt stiff in his low back in the mornings but usually felt looser as the day progressed. He was employed as a tax accountant and was concerned because his busy season was approaching.

Radiographs were ordered by the patient's family physician. Anteroposterior and lateral views revealed moderate degenerative joint disease and degenerative disc disease of the lumbar spine. The physician provided a prescription for Naprosyn, but the patient indicated that he took the medication for only 5 days and then stopped because of stomach irritation.

The patient denied smoking and alcohol abuse. He liked to fly-fish and play cards. He reported that he was in good health other than some mild high blood pressure that was controlled with medication. The patient rated his low back pain as 2 on a scale of 0 to 10. There were no lower extremity symptoms at that time.

What were the important findings from the interview and what could they mean?

The patient's lower extremity symptoms were intermittent and were consistent with activities that involve lumbar extension postures. His mechanism of injury involved repeated lumbar extension (fly-fishing). He attained relief with activities that involved lumbar flexion (sitting, lying in a fetal position). The patient's age (62) and the radiographic findings of degenerative joint disease and degenerative disc disease were consistent with the finding that he was stiff in his low back in the morning and felt less stiff with activity. The adverse reaction the patient had to his medication (Naprosyn) did not allow a determination if he would have obtained adequate relief from taking a nonsteroidal antiinflammatory medication.

PHYSICAL EXAMINATION

What were the key aspects of the physical examination?

The examination began with a postural examination and a lower quarter screen. Those procedures helped to rule out certain sources of the patient's signs and symptoms. They also assisted the examiner to determine what special tests were most appropriate to next perform in the physical examination.[1]

The patient presented with a forward-flexed posture in the lumbar spine. He had a moderate thoracic kyphosis and forward head position. Trunk forward flexion indicated he was able to reach his mid tibia. He appeared to present with tight hamstrings judging from the lack of anterior pelvic rotation during forward flexion. Hypomobility was observed throughout his lumbar spine. He reported stiffness and an increase in low back pain with forward flexion but no reproduction of his lower extremity symptoms. Extension was moderately restricted with a slight increase in his low back pain but no change in his lower extremity symptoms. Side-bending right and left were both moderately restricted with complaints of stiffness but no increase in his lower extremity symptoms.

As a result of the findings (no reproduction of symptoms into the right lower extremity), overpressure was applied with each motion. Overpressures failed to reproduce his distal symptoms but did cause some increase in low back discomfort. Repeated motions were then performed for each motion. Repeated motions indicated that extension and right side-bending reproduced his lower extremity symptoms.[1] A dermatome scan was performed and indicated decreased sensation in the lateral lower leg and dorsum of the foot to the great toe in the L5 dermatome.

Resisted isometrics were performed for hip flexors, knee extensors, knee flexors, ankle dorsiflexors, plantarflexors, and great toe extension. All motions were strong and painless except for ankle dorsiflexion and great toe extension, which were weak and painless. Manual muscle testing of dorsiflexion and great toe extension revealed strength scores of 4/5 in these two muscle groups and 5/5 in all other lower extremity muscle groups. Deep tendon reflexes of the patellar tendon (L4) and calcaneal tendon (S1) were normal.

What were the results of the postural examination and lower quarter screen?

Lumbar flexion appeared to be the patient's posture of choice. His lumbar spine was restricted in all planes of motions, but single motions did not reproduce his distal symptoms. Repeated lumbar extension and side bending toward the right did reproduce his distal symptoms. The results of the resisted isometric testing, manual muscle testing, and sensory testing are indicative of possible L5 nerve root involvement.

What additional special tests helped clarify the meaning of the patient's signs and symptoms?

Passive mobility testing was performed using posterior to anterior (PA) pressures with the patient prone and slightly flexed over a pillow. The testing revealed hypomobility throughout the lumbar spine but demonstrated no reproduction of lower extremity symptoms. Palpable muscle spasm was noted throughout the lumbar erector spinae musculature.

Straight-leg raising was found to be limited to approximately 0 to 65 degrees bilaterally, with complaints of tightness of the hamstring musculature. A lower limb tension test was applied to the sciatic nerve with the patient supine by flexing the hip with the knee extended.[2] This test did not reproduce any lower extremity symptoms. Further tension was applied to the sciatic nerve by adducting and internally rotating the hip and finally dorsiflexing the foot. This test was also negative. A lower limb tension test was applied to the femoral nerve with the patient prone by extending the hip and flexing the knee.[2] (It is important that the lumbar spine be kept in neutral for this test. If the lumbar spine is allowed to extend, then there may be a reproduction of distal symptoms due to a closing of the intervertebral foramen impinging on a nerve root and not from tension of the femoral nerve.) This test was also negative. The patient complained of tightness in the rectus femoris, but reported no paresthesias.

Gait analysis revealed that the patient ambulated in a forward-flexed lumbar spine posture. When asked to ambulate with a more upright posture, he complained of right lower extremity paresthesias after walking approximately 50 feet.

What information was derived from the special tests performed?

Lower limb tension testing determined that applying tension to the sciatic nerve and femoral nerve did not reproduce the patient's symptoms. At the time of the test, it appeared that he did not have impingement of either of these nerves. He was found to have tightness of the hamstrings and rectus femoris muscles. He ambulated with a forward-flexed lumbar posture. Ambulating in an upright, lumbar-extended posture reproduced his symptoms. It appeared that in lumbar extension, with the lumbar intervertebral foramen more closed, the patient would experience his distal symptoms.

What could have been the potential source of the patient's problem?

The patient's history of the onset of his symptoms after fly-fishing led to the possibility that repeated extensions was the possible cause of his back pain and lower extremity paresthesias. Extension also appeared to be involved with the patient's complaint of worsening of his symptoms with standing and walking and easing of the symptoms with sitting and lying in a fetal position. Radiographs showed degenerative joint disease and degenerative disc disease. That finding is often related to lateral spinal stenosis.[3] Additional radiographs of a lateral view in full lumbar extension might have shown the size of the intervertebral foramen was significantly reduced when the lumbar spine was fully extended.

If the patient's lower extremity paresthesias stemmed from inflammation of the nerve root, then there is a strong possibility that he may have gotten some relief from a non-steroidal antiinflammatory drug such as Naprosyn. The patient's reported side effect of stomach irritation, however, is a common problem associated with nonsteroidal antiinflammatory medications.[4]

Because of the patient's history of degenerative joint disease and degenerative disc disease, it was expected that he would have hypomobility with passive mobility testing. The patient ambulated with a flexed lumbar spine because ambulating in extension would have worsened his lower extremity symptoms. The fact that the patient ambulated in forward flexion would cause abnormal stress on the lumbar erector spinae, possibly leading to strain and spasm in these muscles.

Physical examination confirmed that flexion activities worsened his lumbar pain but relieved his paresthesias, whereas extension activities worsened his paresthesias. This finding, along with degenerative disc disease and degenerative joint disease of the lumbar spine, pointed to lateral lumbar spinal stenosis as the primary cause of the patient's symptoms.[5] (Degenerative disc disease, resulting in loss of intervertebral disc height, causes the size of the lumbar intervertebral foramen to become smaller vertically. Degenerative disc disease, resulting in radial bulging of the disc, causes a decrease in the size of the intervertebral foramen from anterior to posterior. Degenerative joint disease of the lumbar zygapophyseal joints of the lumbar spine, resulting in hypertrophy of the joint capsules, causes a decrease in the size of the intervertebral foramen from posterior to anterior. These factors, along with the decreased size of the intervertebral foramen during extension could result in nerve root impingement with lumbar extension.) The patient's signs and symptoms all appeared to involve the right L5 nerve root.

Diagnosis

Physical Therapist Practice Patterns 4F: Impaired Joint Mobility, Motor Function, Muscle Performance, Range of Motion, and

Reflex Integrity Associated with Spinal Disorders and 5F: Impaired Peripheral Nerve Integrity and Muscle Performance Associated with Peripheral Nerve Injury.

Prognosis

GOALS

1. The patient will report decreased low back pain and muscle spasm to 0 on a scale of 0 to 10, so that he may put on his shoes and bend to pick small objects up off the floor without pain in 1 week.
2. The patient will no longer experience pain or paresthesias in the right lower extremity while standing or walking in 3 weeks.
3. The patient will return to pain and paresthesias-free fly-fishing in 6 weeks.

Intervention

The patient was seen for physical therapy four times per week for 4 weeks. Intervention included moist heat and massage to relieve the muscle spasm in the lumbar erector spinae. Gentle flexion exercises were given to stretch the lumbar erector spinae and open the intervertebral foramen. The patient was given a home exercise program of flexion exercises, such as bringing his knees to his chest, trunk curl abdominal strengthening, and posterior pelvic tilt exercises. The knee-to-chest stretching exercises were intended to open the intervertebral foramen and keep pressure off the L5 nerve root. Abdominal strengthening exercises and posterior pelvic tilts were meant to help the patient maintain a posterior pelvic tilt and keep the intervertebral foramen open. The patient was also instructed to avoid forward-flexed postures to relieve stress to the erector spinae and extension

postures, and to avoid impingement of lumbar nerve roots. The patient was instructed to stand and walk in a posterior pelvic tilt. His abdominal strengthening program was progressed to an endurance program.

Once the patient's symptoms were reduced, the patient was instructed in a program to function in a posterior pelvic tilt for all activities to keep his lumbar intervertebral foramen open. This was accomplished by first teaching him to attain the posterior pelvic tilt position and hold it while he changed postures. He was then instructed in other activities, such as standing and walking in that position.

Outcome

The patient's lower extremity pain and paresthesias gradually diminished. He was left with some residual lumbar stiffness that he was able to control with his home exercises and by avoiding sitting for extended periods.

REFERENCES

1. Hertling D, Kessler RM: The lumbosacral-lower limb scan examination. In Hertling D, Kessler RM (eds): *Management of common musculoskeletal disorders* (ed 3), Philadelphia: Lippincott, 1996.
2. McRea R: *Clinical orthopaedic examination* (ed 4), New York: Churchill Livingstone, 1997.
3. McKinnis LN: *Fundamentals of orthopedic radiology*, Philadelphia: FA Davis, 1997.
4. Ciccone CD: *Pharmacology in rehabilitation* (ed 2), Philadelphia: FA Davis, 2002.
5. Fritz JM, Delitto A, Welch WC, Erhard RE: Lumbar spinal stenosis: current concepts in evaluation, management and outcome measurements, *Arch Phys Med Rehabil* 79:700, 1998.

LEARNING OBJECTIVES

The reader will be able to:

1. Discuss reasons to suspect reduced bone density in a selected patient.
2. Identify the need for diagnostic imaging in a patient with a suspected hip fracture.

The reader should know that a 63-year-old obese woman with paraplegia was referred by a family physician to a home health agency for physical therapy. The request was due to a report by the woman's daughter that her mother's right leg was externally rotated and shortened. In addition, the daughter stated that she felt her mother was losing range of motion (ROM) in both lower extremities. The family physician contacted the agency and requested physical therapy examination and intervention. The physician specifically requested ROM and stretching to both lower extremities.

Examination

HISTORY

A review of the patient's past and present medical history revealed that she was obese (5 foot 3 inches and 278 pounds reported) and had hypertension (HTN), an irregular heart rate, congestive heart failure (CHF), nerve pain, osteoporosis, incontinence, and paraplegia. The patient reported a failed spinal surgical procedure approximately 12 years earlier that left her nonambulatory. In discussing the spinal surgery, the patient stated that she was nonambulatory since the surgery, which resulted in motor and sensory impairment in both lower extremities. She also told the physical therapist that it was her understanding that she had suffered a blockage to a spinal artery. On questioning, the patient stated that she had undergone 15 weeks of in-patient rehabilitation after the spinal surgery, with little success. At the time of history-taking, the patient was dependent on a Hoyer lift for all hospital bed-to-chair transfers.

Positioned near the bed was a TV tray, as well as a coffee table on which the patient kept most of her medications. Of the more than 30 tablet bottles, 20 had been prescribed by either the family physician or psychiatrists who had attended to the patient during a recent hospital admission for pneumonia. Among the medications were drugs for HTN (verapamil SR 180), irregular heart rate, and CHF. Pain medication included Neurontin and Tylenol 3 or Oxycodone. Additional medication was identified to treat hyperlipidemia (Lipicor), a thyroid condition (Synthroid), bone demineralization (OsCal), a residual cough (Pertussin HC), and Ditropan to assist in controlling incontinence.

A discussion with both the patient and her daughter revealed that the daughter was the primary caregiver. The daughter revealed that because she was employed part time, her mother was home alone approximately 4 to 6 hours per day, 3 days per week. The daughter said that since her mother had a urinary catheter, the only time she had to be moved was for bowel movements, for which a bedpan was used. The daughter also said that her mother was moved out of bed, via a Hoyer lift, two to three times a week for sponge baths, performed in the living room with towels on the floor.

SYSTEMS REVIEW

Vital signs were measured and found to be within normal limits.

What specific tests and measures were appropriate for this patient?

TESTS AND MEASURES

Musculoskeletal assessment revealed decreased but functional ROM in both upper extremities. ROM was mildly limited secondary to pain at both shoulders and was attributed to recently diagnosed left shoulder bursitis and right shoulder impingement syndrome. Muscle strength in both upper extremities was good to good+ throughout. The left lower extremity had passive ROM within functional limits throughout. Tightness was noted in the hip flexors and hamstring musculature. The right lower extremity appeared flexed and externally rotated.

Passive ROM (PROM) of the left hip and knee were noted to be within functional limits. A left ankle PROM limitation was noted in dorsiflexion, lacking 15 degrees from neutral. Strength testing of the left lower extremity was poor to poor+ throughout (the patient was able to elicit weak muscle contractions throughout). At the hip, the patient was unable to perform a straight leg raise, complete hip abduction, or internally rotate from a fully externally rotated position to neutral. At the knee, the patient was unable to complete terminal knee extension or flexion and had incomplete active movement in both plantarflexion and dorsiflexion.

The right lower extremity position (at rest) was observed and recorded as follows: hip flexion approximately 20 degrees, hip external rotation approximately 30 degrees, and knee flexion approximately 50 degrees. The patient denied any pain in the groin, hip, or buttock area with palpation. She reported a greater degree of difficulty moving the right leg versus the left. She also commented that the right leg felt heavier and the hip tighter and stiff.

Sensory testing resulted in reported deficits throughout the right lower extremity, with no consistency in dermatomes when compared with the left leg. The patient reiterated the presence of occasional "nerve pain" in both legs and feet.

What action was appropriate for the therapist to take?

Evaluation

The patient's hip position, as well as her past medical history, were of concern to the physical therapist. Because the list of possible problems included a fractured hip, the therapist contacted the agency nurse who had completed the home care admission. That nurse stated that although she had some "concerns" regarding the patient's hip position, she kept in mind the patient's past history and litany of complaints, as well as the fact that the patient had stated that the physical therapist was scheduled to come in later that afternoon. The therapist suggested that there was a suspicion of a hip fracture.

Diagnosis

Insufficient information gathered during the physical therapy examination to enable identification of a specific practice pattern from the *Guide to Physical Therapist Practice*.

Intervention

The therapist contacted the referring physician, requesting that radiographs be taken of the patient's right hip. The physician stated that although he had ordered numerous radiographs of this patient over the past 12 to 15 months for "suspected" problems, he would heed the therapist's advice and order a mobile radiograph.

A follow-up telephone call to the physician's office the next day confirmed the presence of an oblique fracture through the surgical neck of the right hip. It was explained that the physician, although surprised, wanted to extend his appreciation for the therapist's phone call the previous day.

Outcome and Discussion

In this case, the patient's history was complex and necessitated a complete physical examination by the physical therapist. Given the position of the right lower extremity and the patient's history of relative immobility, the therapist wisely suspected hip pathology. Correctly, the therapist recommended diagnostic imaging.

Having received a definitive diagnosis from the physician, the physical therapist discussed the case with two orthopedic surgeons. After hearing specifics of the case, both of these surgeons agreed that the patient was not a good surgical candidate, and if they were consulted, they would treat the patient conservatively. Both suggested that the hip not receive ROM or be stretched for at least 4 to 6 weeks or until radiographs showed sufficient callus formation to ensure stability and strength of the hip.

RECOMMENDED READINGS

Kottke FJ, Lehmann JF: *Krusen's handbook of physical medicine and rehabilitation* (ed 4), Philadelphia: WB Saunders, 1990.

Hertling D, Kessler RM: *Management of common musculoskeletal disorders* (ed 3), Philadelphia: Lippincott, 1996.

Magee DJ: *Orthopedic physical assessment* (ed 3), Philadelphia: WB Saunders, 1997.

Fagerson TL: *The hip handbook*, Oxford, UK: Butterworth-Heinemann, 1998.

Case 25

LEARNING OBJECTIVES

The reader will be able to:

1. Identify the need for referral to other health care providers.
2. Recognize abnormal findings on an exercise stress test.
3. Develop a plan of treatment for a patient in inpatient and outpatient cardiac rehabilitation.
4. Identify patient education issues related to cardiac surgery.

The reader should know that the patient was a 61-year-old female referred to an outpatient physical therapy clinic with the diagnosis of "back pain—evaluate and treat." She went to her family physician with a complaint of back pain when walking for a long time and when doing household chores. The pain was "mainly between the shoulder blades."

Examination and Evaluation

The physical therapy examination was unremarkable, and symptoms were not reproduced. The patient's personal medical history included high cholesterol levels, a cholecystectomy performed in 1993, postmenopausal for 7-years, and a family history of heart disease (her mother died at age 61 of a myocardial infarction [MI]). The patient did not participate in any recreational activity at the time.

Based on a lack of clinical findings, what would be an appropriate course of action for the therapist to take?

The patient was referred back to her family doctor with the results of the physical therapy examination and history. The therapist suggested that because the patient's pain was not reproduced and heart disease was a component of her family history, that a cardiopulmonary assessment be performed. The physician ordered an exercise stress test (EST), which yielded a 3-mm ST segment depression in leads V_5 and V_6, and her systolic

blood pressure dropped 22 mm Hg at stage III of the Bruce protocol treadmill test.

Of what significance were those EST findings?

Back pain from the history is a sign of coronary artery disease (CAD). Women are twice as likely as men to describe back pain as a symptom before acute MI. The EST yielded a 3-mm ST segment depression in leads V_5 and V_6, which is indicative of ischemia. Because this occurred in leads V_5 and V_6, the left anterior descending and circumflex arteries should be evaluated for stenosis. In addition, the patient experienced a drop in systolic blood pressure during exercise. This "exercise-induced hypotension" (drop in systolic blood pressure with an increase in work rate) is seen in individuals with CAD, valvar heart disease, cardiomyopathies, and dysrhythmias. It is correlated with myocardial ischemia and left ventricular dysfunction.

The patient was referred to a cardiologist, who ordered a cardiac catheterization. Based on the findings, the cardiologist recommended coronary artery bypass graft (CABG) surgery. One day after the CABG, done via a median sternotomy approach, the patient was seen by a physical therapist in the intensive care unit. She had a chest tube on her left side, a temporary pacemaker, an arterial line in her right upper extremity, and an arterial oxygen saturation monitor on her right index finger. Further, she was connected to a 12-lead electrocardiogram (ECG) monitor. Her resting

109

vital signs were blood pressure, 132/82 mm Hg; heart rate, 88 beats per minute (bpm); and respiratory rate, 16 breaths per minute; oxygen saturation on room air was 96%. The patient was referred for inpatient (also known as phase I) cardiac rehabilitation. Assuming no complications, the patient was scheduled for discharge to home on postoperative day 5.

Diagnosis

Physical Therapist Practice Pattern 6D: Impaired Aerobic Capacity/Endurance Associated with Cardiovascular Pump Dysfunction or Failure.

Intervention

If an assumption was made that the patient planned to return home, what plan of progression—when to get out of bed, ambulate, ascend/descend steps—and what type of therapeutic exercise would be recommended? What patient education issues existed?

The plan of care for postoperative cardiac surgery generally follows a "step" program or an "activity classification." Excluding any postoperative complications, her acute care length of stay would likely be 4 to 6 days. It is critical that early mobilization occur. Most of the hemodynamic monitoring lines (e.g., Swan-Ganz catheter) were discontinued by postoperative day 1. The patient was monitored either by a bedside ECG unit or by telemetry throughout the hospital stay. When the patient was hemodynamically stable, postoperative day 1 activity included being out of bed to a chair and sitting up in the chair for 15 to 30 minutes. She also performed active ROM (AROM) cardinal plane therapeutic exercise while seated, as well as deep-breathing exercises, incentive spirometry, and splinted coughing. On postoperative days 2 and 3, the patient was progressed to out of bed to a chair three times per day and continued therapeutic exercise in sitting or standing positions. The patient generally walked up to 50 to 100 feet, and patient education focused on sternal precautions,

avoiding the Valsalva maneuver, and risk factor modification. On postoperative days 4 to 6, the patient walked more than 200 feet and ascended and descended steps. In this case, an exercise tolerance test was performed before the patient was discharged. Patient education focused on guidelines for a safe and effective home exercise program (HEP) and a discussion about outpatient cardiac rehabilitation.

What were some HEP considerations?

Guidelines for safe activity in the acute care program and the HEP will vary depending on such factors as medications and results of exercise testing. In general, patients should be asymptomatic, with a heart rate limited to resting rate plus <30 bpm. Clinicians often use the rating of perceived exertion (RPE) scale to judge appropriate intensity, which is useful for patients taking medication that blunts their heart rate (e.g., beta blockers). An RPE of <13 is recommended. The HEP should be geared toward increasing activity, with a goal of achieving 10 to 15 minutes of continued ambulation. Therapeutic exercise should continue with cardinal plane AROM without resistance. Patient education should focus on avoiding prolonged overhead reaching, which will increase stress on the healing sternum and also place additional workload on the heart.

The patient spent 5 days in the hospital and was then discharged to home. Six weeks after undergoing CABG surgery, she was referred to outpatient cardiac rehabilitation (also known as phase II and III).

Should the physical therapist prescribe resistance exercises? If so, what exercise prescription—type of exercise, frequency, intensity, repetitions/sets, and any precautions—would be discussed with the patient?

Resistance exercise was an integral part of this patient's cardiac rehabilitation program. Light Theraband and cuff weights (1 to 3 pounds) were initiated early in the outpatient program. However, traditional strength training was delayed until 3 months after the sternotomy, and the sternum was assessed for stability by an experienced health care provider before initiating weight training. In general, patients participate in outpatient cardiac rehabilitation focusing on increasing aerobic functional capacity for 6 weeks before initiating resistance training. During and after the 6 weeks of aerobic training, the patient was educated on avoiding the Valsalva maneuver and performed baseline strength training, with a one-repetition maximum (1-RM) program. Resistance exercise focused on major muscle groups (quadriceps, hamstrings, chest/back, and arms). The resistance was set at approximately 40% of 1-RM and the patient performed 8 to 15 repetitions in 1 to 3 sets for 3 nonconsecutive days per week. All exercises were done in a slow, controlled manner without breath holding. To adhere to RPE guidelines, the 1-RM was reevaluated every 2 weeks, and adjustments to the weight load were made.

Outcome

The patient completed 36 sessions of outpatient treatment over 3 months. On discharge, the patient was independent in recalling her cardiac risk factors and able to complete 40 minutes of continuous aerobic exercise 4 days per week. She also performed a circuit weight-training program consisting of four lower body and five upper body exercises using variable-resistance isotonic machines and dumbbells. She understood the importance of adding resistance, and by the end of the 3 months was performing 60% of her 1-RM for 2 sets of 8 to 15 repetitions for each of the exercises on 3 nonconsecutive days. She immediately joined a local health club to continue the exercise program as a means of preventing future cardiac problems and to improve overall health.

RECOMMENDED READINGS

ACSM: *Guidelines for exercise testing and prescription* (ed 6), Baltimore: Williams & Wilkins, 2000.

American Heart Association: Science advisory: resistance exercise in individuals with and without cardiovascular disease, *Circulation* 101:828, 2000.

Beniamini Y, Rubenstein JJ, Faigenbaum AD, et al: High intensity strength training of patients enrolled in an outpatient cardiac rehabilitation program, *J Cardiopulm Rehabil* 19:8, 1999.

Hillegass EA, Sadowsky HS: *Essentials of cardiopulmonary physical therapy* (ed 2), Philadelphia: WB Saunders, 2001.

Verrill DE, Ribisl PM: Resistive exercise training in cardiac rehabilitation: an update, *Sports Med* 21:347, 1996.

LEARNING OBJECTIVES

The reader will be able to:

1. Identify the appropriate rehabilitation management strategy (physical therapy and prosthetic assessments, interventions, and follow-up) for a child with traumatic amputation over the continuum of his care.

2. Describe how cognitive and behavioral recovery after traumatic brain injury may affect prosthetic rehabilitation.

3. Incorporate understanding of a child and a family's response to a life-altering traumatic event into a physical therapy plan of care.

4. In a multidisciplinary team, select the appropriate prosthetic components from among available options, and determine the effectiveness of prosthetic fit and alignment (static and dynamic).

5. Discuss the collaborative roles of outpatient and school-based physical therapy in facilitating a child's return to the educational setting after traumatic amputation.

Examination

HISTORY

The patient was a 7-year-old boy who was 5 weeks status post multiple traumatic injuries sustained in late September in a car–bicycle accident on the street in front of his home. He suffered severe crush injuries of the distal lower extremities, closed-head injury, ruptured spleen, and multiple abrasions. He was flown by medical helicopter to the regional pediatric trauma center, a 45-minute drive from his home. In the emergency room, his Glasgow coma score was 9 (eye opening, 3 to speech; best motor response, 4 withdraws; verbal response, 2 incomprehensible sounds). On further evaluation of his condition in the emergency room, the trauma team determined that amputation and splenectomy were necessary. In the intensive care unit (ICU) after surgery, the patient's breathing was supported by synchronized intermittent mandatory ventilation (SIMV) for 24 hours while he was kept sedated. Postoperatively, a course of intravenous broad-spectrum antibiotics was started to reduce the risk of infection of his residual limbs.

After 5 days in the ICU, the patient was transferred to the pediatric rehabilitation unit for cognitive status assessment, functional mobility training, and preprosthetic assessment. He was discharged to home with a wheelchair and appropriate adaptive equipment in mid-October, after a 3-week hospital stay. After discharge, he returned to the hospital for continued rehabilitation on an outpatient basis three times per week. His initial prostheses were fitted and delivered, and early prosthetic training begun. He prepared to return to school in mid-November. He continued with functional prosthetic training on an outpatient setting and was scheduled for evaluation by the school-based physical therapist to facilitate reentry into school-related activities.

Before his injuries, the patient was a healthy and active 7-year-old, the oldest of three children in his family. His mother worked at home as a graphic artist for an advertising agency, and his father commuted by train to his office job in a nearby city. The patient was in the second grade at his suburban elementary school and was an active participant in the town's soccer and baseball leagues. He also had been active in Cub Scouts and particularly enjoyed woodworking activities. The family lived in a two-storey home with bedrooms and a full bathroom upstairs. The home had three steps, with no railings, to enter the house from either the garage or front door entries.

SYSTEMS REVIEW

Cognitive status. When the patient returned home, he was functioning at Rancho Los Amigos cognitive level 7, automatic-appropriate, demonstrating mild distractibility, mild emotional lability with reduced tolerance to challenging or stressful situations, mild learning/memory impairment, and some difficulty with problem solving, planning, and organization skills. Language comprehension and expression were intact. Although the patient was anxious to regain his independence and walk with his prostheses, he relied heavily on the encouragement and support of his parents and therapists. He often displayed anxiety about falling and quickly sought outside assistance from his caregivers in activities that he perceived to be overly challenging in terms of his standing balance. His frustration level fluctuated, and his desire to return to soccer or baseball was a motivational tool at times. His emerging sense of self when compared with classmates helped to raise his anxiety about returning to school. He resisted the idea of using his wheelchair at school and had several outbursts related to this issue.

Neurologic status. The mild to moderate vestibular impairment present during the patient's early in-patient rehabilitation resolved. No other residual neurologic impairments were noted, although deep tendon reflexes at the quadriceps were brisk. The patient's awareness of limb position in space at the hip and knee appeared to be intact. Somatosensation (pain, temperature, and touch) was also intact, except in areas of split-thickness skin grafts on the lateral thigh and knee of the right residual limb. He had mild paresthesias with some hypersensitivity adjacent to the suture line bilaterally. He reported fairly consistent phantom sensation (deep cramping in the calf on the left, itchy toes on the right) that decreased in intensity when compression garments were reapplied.

Integumentary status.
The patient's splenectomy incision was well healed, as were the abrasions on his face, arms, and trunk. There was a healed 2- × 4-inch split-thickness skin graft (used to close deep abrasion) on the right lateral thigh and knee, as well as a well-healed donor site on the left anterior thigh.

The patient had a standard-length (5-inch) posterior flap transtibial amputation on the right. In his early prosthetic training, a quarter-inch area of dehiscence (with slight serosanguinous drainage) developed at the most-medial suture line; it was held closed with Steri-Strips. His surgical scar otherwise healed well and was mobile, with no obvious areas of adhesion. His residual limb was well shaped, with no redundant tissue. He had a short (3-inch) "fish mouth" closure transtibial amputation on the left. There was a "dimple" skin fold 1½ inches from the lateral edge of his incision. The incision healed well, was mobile, and had no obvious areas of adhesion. There was an area of persistent redness over the distal anterior residual tibia.

What types of measurable data should be gathered?

Volume control and protection of both residual limbs was managed with compressive shrinker garments (to mid-thigh) and removable rigid dressings (which he required assistance to don). Circumferential measurements of limbs (supine, with knee extended) were as follows:

- 2 inches above the proximal border of the patella: 14.75 inches in the left lower extremity (LLE); 14.50 inches in the right lower extremity (RLE)
- At the proximal border of the patella: 13.25 inches in the LLE; 13.00 inches in the RLE
- At the distal border of the patella: 13.00 inches in the LLE; 13.00 inches in the RLE
- At the proximal tibial tubercle: 13.25 inches in the LLE; 13.00 inches in the RLE
- 2 inches below the tibial tubercle: 13.50 inches in the LLE; 13.25 inches in the RLE
- 4 inches below the tibial tubercle: 13.25 inches in the RLE

Strength and muscle performance. Strength and muscle performance ratings were as follows:

- Upper extremities: 4 to 4+ throughout, bilaterally
- Trunk: gross abdominal strength 4
- Hip flexion, adduction, and rotation: 4 bilaterally
- Hip extension and abduction: 4– bilaterally
- Knee: LLE extension 4, flexion 4–; RLE extension 3+, flexion 3+

Joint function and range of motion. On examination, all ligaments of the LLE were intact. Mild instability of the medial collateral ligament of the RLE was noted. There were flexion contractures (5 degrees LLE, 8 degrees RLE) with firm end feels. The patient was able to actively flex to 120 degrees in the LLE and to 105 degrees in the RLE. Active excursion of straight leg raise was 95 degrees in the LLE and 85 degrees in the RLE.

Endurance. The patient described a rate of perceived exertion of 7 during ambulation activities and 9 during stair-climbing activities. Mild deconditioning was noted with an increased respiratory rate of 24 breaths per minute (bpm) during ambulation (baseline rate, 21 bpm at rest).

Postural control. Static postural control and anticipatory postural changes were intact in sitting in all directions. Equilibrium reactions and protective responses appeared to be intact in static sitting, with occasional loss of balance (backward) with moderately forceful perturbation in the long sitting or short sitting position (without prosthesis). His forward reach distance in short sitting was more than 10 inches, and his lateral reach in short sitting was 8 inches to the left and 7 inches to the right.

The patient was able to stand unsupported on his prostheses for up to 30 seconds; however, he preferred at least unilateral upper extremity support to allay his anxiety about falling. In the parallel bars, he was able to independently step forward and shift his weight between the anterior and posterior foot. He was hesitant to step unsupported outside of parallel bars, preferring bilateral Loftstrand crutches or straight canes.

How might this child access his home environment?

Functional mobility. The patient used a rented Quickie wheelchair for mobility at home. The chair was fitted with long anti-tippers to accommodate the changes in his center of mass resulting from the amputations. He became independent in wheelchair mobility on level surfaces and slight inclines but required minimal to moderate assistance for propulsion on uneven surfaces and grades greater than 15 degrees. He also became independent in most level transfers (bed, toilet, and bath bench) and used a transfer board with minimal assistance for car transfers. He preferred to be lifted to and from the floor, but was able to perform chair-to-floor transfers with verbal cues and minimal assistance.

After gait training, the patient used a four-point reciprocal gait pattern with Lofstrand crutches, with close supervision when on level uncarpeted surfaces for distances up to 150 feet between skin checks. He was able to ascend stairs step to step leading with the left leg, using a crutch and handrail and contact guard assistance. He was fearful when descending, requiring verbal encouragement, minimal assistance, and occasional correction of balance.

Adaptive equipment and assistive devices. Both prostheses were fabricated with endoskeletal (modular) components, with flexible polyvinyl patellar tendon-bearing sockets in rigid polyethylene frames. They had shuttle pin suspension mechanisms, based on an Ortho Gel (roll-on) liner (Figure 26-1). To don the prosthesis, the patient steps down (clicks down) into the prosthesis to engage the shuttle-locking mechanism. Suspension was released by an external release positioned on the medial-distal frame of the prosthesis. Initially, he had a pair of Seattle dynamic response prosthetic feet.

How might fluctuating limb volume be accommodated?

The patient wore a five-ply cotton sock (with a hole cut for the pin) over the right Ortho

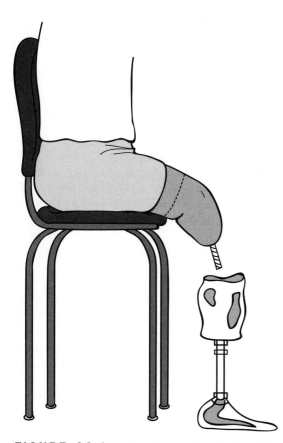

FIGURE 26-1 To don his prosthesis, the child first rolls the Ortho Gel liner with embedded locking pin directly over the skin of his residual limb. He then applies prosthetic socks (with a distal opening for the pin) over the liner. He sits on the edge of the chair, positions his limb in the socket, and steps down (clicks down) to engage the shuttle-locking mechanism. (Used with permission.)

Gel liner, and a five-ply wool sock (with a hole cut for the pin) on the left. His mother carried additional one-ply cotton socks to adjust for volume changes as his activity increased.

Bench and static alignment. To accommodate for knee flexion contractures, the socket was set (preflexed) at 10 degrees on the right and 12 degrees on the left. There was a 5-degree lateral tilt of both sockets. His prosthetic feet were aligned a ¾-inch outset with respect to the socket. On the right, the prosthetic foot was placed in a neutral position, whereas the left prosthetic

foot was positioned slightly anterior (¼ inch) to enhance knee extensor moment for stability at midstance. When the prostheses were doffed after a period of quiet standing, there was appropriate reactive hyperemia in expected pressure-tolerant areas, although there was moderate persistent redness at the right distal tibia.

Dynamic alignment. Observational gait analysis revealed a slightly wide step width, moderately shortened stride and step lengths, and increased double support time. Walking velocity was somewhat slow, apparently related to the patient's apprehension about falling. As a result, he was not effectively using the dynamic response characteristics of late stance/transition to the swing phase. With encouragement, he was able to increase stride length and velocity. He complained of feeling as if his left knee was being pushed into extension as he moved into midstance. Toe clearance was adequate in early swing, although he tended to limit knee flexion in initial swing phase, resulting in a slightly stiff-legged gait. With encouragement, he was able to step over obstacles up to 3 inches in height. When asked to identify where he felt pressure on his residual limbs when he stood and walked, he pointed to a large area of the medial tibial flare and the distal lateral surface of the tibia, as well as at the insertion of the patellar tendon. He indicated that the sockets felt "tight," but there were no areas of point tenderness.

Diagnosis

PRIMARY

Physical Therapy Practice Pattern 4J: Impaired Motor Function, Muscle Performance, Range of Motion, Gait, Locomotion, and Balance Associated with Amputation.

SECONDARY

Physical Therapy Practice Pattern 5C: Impaired Motor Function, and Sensory Integrity Associated with Nonprogressive Disorders of the Central Nervous System—Congenital in Origin or Acquired in Infancy or Childhood.

Prognosis

GOALS

1. The patient will return to his elementary school environment and participate as fully as possible in school-related activities within 2 months.
2. The patient will return to valued leisure activities, or find appropriate alternative/adaptive activities, and participate as fully as possible within 6 months.

EXPECTED OUTCOMES

1. The patient and his parents will demonstrate effective and consistent skin care and volume control strategies as his residual limbs mature.
2. The patient and his parents will demonstrate proper donning/doffing of prosthesis; he will wear the prostheses functionally for most of the day.
3. Muscle performance (strength), ROM, and postural control and balance will improve. The patient will demonstrate full ROM and 5/5 in his lower extremities. He will perform the one-legged stance test for 30 seconds without losing his balance while wearing the prostheses on both his right and left limbs. He will be able to maintain semitandem and tandem Romberg positions for 25 seconds.
4. Cognitive function will improve and/or he will develop appropriate adaptive strategies necessary for effective return to school and leisure activities.
5. Prosthetic gait and functional mobility skills will be safe, efficient, and functional for home, school, and leisure activities, as evidenced by improved scores on the dynamic gait index and gait assessment rating scale (GARS).
6. The patient will resume full participation in his previous or adapted recreational activities.

DISCHARGE PLAN

Mechanisms of communication between outpatient and school-based care were established. The patient was discharged from outpatient physical therapy when there was consensus among outpatient physical thera-pists, prosthetists, parents, and the patient that he had achieved functional goals for effective community reentry (considering both amputation/prosthetic and traumatic brain injury rehabilitation). He received school-based physical therapy for the school year, and was scheduled for reevaluation in September as the next school year began to determine whether continued school-based physical therapy was necessary. Based on anticipated periods of growth, the patient was enrolled for long-term follow-up (post-discharge) at the interdisciplinary prosthetics clinic at the children's hospital.

Intervention

The following interventions were implemented:
1. Continue gait training and advanced mobility training as an outpatient, with the goals of improving musculoskeletal function, quality of gait, functional mobility skills, and functional endurance.
2. Pursue school-based physical therapy services and special education services to ensure appropriate reentry into school.
3. Identify strategies for periodic reevaluation to determine progression (and/or barriers) toward functional goals and effective community reentry.
4. Set up a mechanism for communication/collaboration between outpatient-based and school-based physical therapy services.
5. Identify current and project future needs for adaptation of (or assistive devices) in home, school, and leisure activities.
6. Monitor the effectiveness of the prosthetic prescription; consider alternative components and transition to "permanent" prostheses when appropriate (taking into consideration anticipated growth).

Outcome (3 months after returning to school)

When the patient first returned to school, his behavior indicated mildly compromised function in particularly complex, stimulating, active, or unpredictable environments. There was, however, nearly complete resolution of most cognitive impairments related to his head injury in the 3 months after his return to school. He became actively and effectively involved in classroom and playground activities. Although alternative physical education activities were made available, he became anxious to rejoin his buddies in regular "gym" class.

During that 3-month period, the patient made significant progress in functional mobility and ambulation. Currently, he walks without any assistive devices on level surfaces at school and home, and keeps up with his classmates in both distance covered and energy cost of walking. He prefers to use a single cane on the right side when weather conditions make environmental surfaces slippery; other times his cane becomes a "Jedi light saber" during imaginative play. He now manages stairs in a step-over-step pattern using one rail. He has experienced several noninjurious falls during playground and gym activities, is able to rise independently, and no longer worries about falling. He dons his prostheses independently in the morning, wears them all day, and often removes them in late afternoon to actively play on the floor with his sisters.

He is looking forward to playing "T-ball" this spring, although members of the town's recreation department have expressed some hesitation about the appropriateness of his involvement; he is the first child with amputation who wants to be involved in the program.

He is now wearing 15-ply wool socks over his suspension sleeve on both residual limbs; at his last visit to prosthetic clinic, the team began to discuss whether it is time to fabricate new prosthetic sockets. As a result of increasing activity and consistent stretching, he has regained full extension of both knees, which has necessitated several adjustments to alignment of prosthetic components. He currently visits the outpatient rehabilitation department once weekly; activities focus on advanced mobility skills and leisure activities.

RECOMMENDED READINGS

Auxter D, Pyfer J, Huettig C: *Principles and methods of adapted physical education and recreation* (ed 9), New York: McGraw Hill, 2001.

Berke GM: Transtibial prosthetics. In Lusardi MM, Nielsen CC (eds): *Orthotics & prosthetics in rehabilitation*, Boston: Butterworth-Heinemann, 2000.

Both A: Traumatic brain injury in childhood. In Tecklin JS (ed): *Pediatric physical therapy* (ed 3), New York: Lippincott Williams & Wilkins, 1999.

Edelstein JE: Rehabilitation for children with limb deficiencies. In Lusardi MM, Nielsen CC (eds): *Orthotics & prosthetics in rehabilitation*, Boston: Butterworth-Heinemann, 2000.

Effgen SK: The educational environment. In Campbell SK, Vander Linden DW, Palisano RJ (eds): *Physical therapy for children* (ed 2), Philadelphia: WB Saunders, 2000.

Fergusen J: Prosthetic feet. In Lusardi MM, Nielsen CC (eds): *Orthotics & prosthetics in rehabilitation*, Boston: Butterworth-Heinemann, 2000.

Keirkering GA, Phillips W: Brain injuries: traumatic brain injuries, near-drowning, and brain tumors. In Campbell SK, Vander Linden DW, Palisano RJ (eds): *Physical therapy for children* (ed 2), Philadelphia: WB Saunders, 2000.

Lunnen KY: Physical therapy in public schools. In Tecklin JS (ed): *Pediatric physical therapy* (ed 3), New York: Lippincott Williams & Wilkins, 1999.

Lusardi MM, Owens LF: Post-operative and pre-prosthetic care. In Lusardi MM, Nielsen CC (eds): *Orthotics & prosthetics in rehabilitation*, Boston: Butterworth-Heinemann, 2000.

May BJ: *Amputations and prosthetics: a case study approach*, Philadelphia: FA Davis, 1996.

American Physical Therapy Association. McEwen I (ed): Providing physical therapy services under parts b & c of the Individuals with Disabilities Act (IDEA). Section on Pediatrics, 2000.

Reis JD, Brewer KM: Transtibial prosthetic training and rehabilitation. In Lusardi MM, Nielsen CC (eds): *Orthotics & prosthetics in rehabilitation*, Boston: Butterworth-Heinemann, 2000.

Seymour R: *Prosthetics & orthotics: lower limb and spinal*, Philadelphia: Lippincott Williams & Wilkins, 2002.

Stanger M: Limb deficiencies and amputations. In Campbell SK, Vander Linden DW, Palisano RJ (eds): *Physical therapy for children* (ed 2), Philadelphia: WB Saunders, 2000.

Stanger M: Orthopedic management. In Tecklin JS (ed): *Pediatric physical therapy* (ed 3), New York: Lippincott Williams & Wilkins, 2000.

Winkler PA: Traumatic brain injuries. In Umphred DA (ed): *Neurological rehabilitation* (ed 4), St Louis: Mosby, 2001.

Winnick JP (ed): *Adapted physical education and sport* (ed 3), Champaign, Ill, Human Kinetics, 2000.

LEARNING OBJECTIVES

The reader will be able to:

1. Describe how the results of medical imaging may affect a physical therapy plan of care.
2. Describe how psychosocial issues such as depression may affect both the physical therapy plan of care and the patient's long-term outcome.
3. Discuss factors one must consider when planning a treatment for a patient with multiple chronic conditions.
4. Discuss whether patients can benefit from the use of constraint-induced movement therapy as part of a plan of care to promote improved gait.

Examination

HISTORY

The patient was a 40-year-old woman who worked full time as a social worker in a rehabilitation hospital. She had right-sided hemiparesis caused by a left anterior cerebral artery aneurysm sustained 20 years earlier. Her right leg was more affected than her right arm. She had spasticity in both extremities and had right finger flexor contractures that limited the use of her hand. She was previously right-hand dominant, but now used her left hand for most functional activities (e.g., writing, grooming, hygiene). She used her right hand functionally as an assist. She was 5 feet, 8 inches tall and weighed 190 pounds.

The patient had significant baseline gait deviations with a subsequent history of back and neck pain. She used a single-point cane for all gait activities; she was independent in mobility on all surfaces indoors and outdoors. She lived alone in a second-story apartment. There were five steps to enter the building, and there was no elevator.

On February 20, the patient tripped and fell in her apartment. She noted pain and swelling in her left knee. Despite the pain, she attempted to continue with her daily activities. One week later, she continued to have pain and swelling of the left knee. On February 27, she was seen by her primary care physician, who diagnosed a sprain of the right medial collateral ligament. Because of the degree of pain and swelling, a radiograph was ordered. Results were negative for fracture.

The physician recommended restricted weight bearing because of pain and swelling. The physician also recommended using an ace wrap to reduce swelling, and an antiinflammatory drug for pain and swelling. Because of the weakness in her right arm and leg, the patient had difficulty maintaining the partial weight-bearing restrictions. The physician ordered a physical therapy consult to address the problem.

What tests and measures were important to include in the initial examination?

What recommendations could have been made for this patient in terms of an assistive device?

Which practice pattern(s) in the Guide to Physical Therapist Practice would be appropriate for this patient?

What other physical therapy intervention(s), if any, could be recommended?

INITIAL EXAMINATION

Date: March 1

The physical therapist performed the following tests and measures.

Pain. The patient described the pain in her knee as a 7 out of 10, worsening to a 9 out of 10 at the end of the day.

Peripheral nerve integrity, muscle performance and sensory integrity. *Sensation:* Sensation was intact throughout the left side, and decreased on the right side, with the right leg more affected than the right arm. Proprioception, kinesthesia, and sharp/dull testing were decreased in the right leg.

Strength: Because of the spasticity present on the right side, the physical therapist did not assign manual muscle test grades. The left arm was functional throughout. The left hip and ankle had functional strength; because of pain, left knee strength was not tested.

The patient was able to elevate the right arm about 45 degrees. Elbow flexion was functional. She was able to fully extend her elbow in a gravity-eliminated position and extend her elbow about 30 degrees against gravity. She had minimal motion in her right wrist and hand. Her wrist rested in neutral, and her hand rested in a clawed position. She was unable to carry objects in the right hand.

The patient was able to flex the right hip against gravity about 20 degrees with maximal effort. She tended to substitute by using back extension. She was able to extend the right hip fully against gravity but could not accept resistance to the movement. When she attempted to abduct the hip in standing, she tended to lean toward her left side. Without leaning, she demonstrated minimal abduction against gravity. When supine, she was able to abduct her hip about 45 degrees. She was able to extend her right knee fully against gravity and could accept minimal resistance. Increased resistance caused increased extensor tone throughout. She had minimal movement in ankle dorsiflexion and no active ankle plantarflexion.

Range of motion. The left side was functional; because of pain, the left knee was not tested. The right shoulder had decreased passive range of motion in shoulder elevation and external rotation. The wrist and fingers had limited motion in all planes. The right leg was functional except for ankle dorsiflexion and plantarflexion, which were both limited to 10 degrees.

Posture. The patient sat and stood with a slight posterior pelvic tilt, with more weight on the left side. The trunk was rotated forward on the left. The right shoulder was lower than the left. Slight forward head was present.

Gait, locomotion, and balance. The patient had been using a single-point cane for all gait. She took a short step with the right foot, because of the left knee pain. Because of weakness, she also took a small step with the left foot. Other gait deviations included right knee extension throughout the entire gait cycle, right hip hiking and circumduction, and decreased weight shifting onto the right leg.

The physical therapist tested the patient's static and dynamic balance using the Tinetti assessment tool and the Berg balance scale. The patient scored 18 out of a possible 28 points on the Tinetti assessment tool and 33 out of a possible 56 on the Berg balance scale. Both indicated that she was at risk for future falls. Although both scales were designed for the elderly, the physical therapist decided to use them to provide baseline measurements of the patient's dynamic balance.

Assistive and adaptive devices. The patient attempted to use a large base quad cane but was unable to adequately unweight her left leg to achieve a partial weight-bearing gait. Because of the weakness in her right arm and leg, the patient was unable to use crutches.

Evaluation

After the examination, the physical therapist recommended a wheeled walker with a right upper extremity platform. The decision was based on several factors, including the strength available in the patient's extremities and the patient's ability to successfully decrease the amount of weight that she put through her left leg.

Although the patient was concerned about the bulkiness of the wheeled walker, she agreed to use it. Her biggest concern was that it would be difficult for her to get the walker up to her second-floor apartment. She and the therapist practiced having the patient fold the walker and carry it up the stairs. She was able to do it but reported that the activity was very fatiguing.

Diagnosis

The physical therapist classified this patient under two different practice patterns, because of the complexity of her history. First, the physical therapist chose Pattern 4D: Impaired Joint Mobility, Motor Function, Muscle Performance, and Range of Motion Associated with Connective Tissue Dysfunction. This pattern includes patients with ligamentous sprain, pain, and swelling. The expected range of visits for this pattern is between 3 and 36.

The physical therapist also chose Pattern 5D: Impaired Motor Function and Sensory Integrity Associated with Nonprogressive Disorders of the Central Nervous System— Acquired in Adolescence or Adulthood. This pattern includes patients who have had a cerebrovascular accident and who have impaired motor function. It also includes difficulty negotiating terrains and inability to perform work activities, both of which were potential problems for the patient. The expected range of visits for this pattern is 10 to 60.

Prognosis

Because of the patient's significant past medical history, the therapist predicted that she might need a longer course than usual for rehabilitation. At the time, the physical therapist felt that the patient needed to concentrate on resting her injured left leg by minimizing weight-bearing during gait. The therapist believed that the patient needed to improve the strength of her right arm and leg to allow her to rest her left leg.

GOALS

1. The patient will maintain partial weight-bearing gait for the left lower extremity on all surfaces using a wheeled platform walker independently in 2 weeks.
2. The patient will extend her right elbow 60 degrees against gravity to allow improved support while using a walker in 2 weeks.

3. The patient will flex her right hip 40 degrees against gravity to improve her ability to advance her right leg during gait in 2 weeks.
4. The patient will demonstrate understanding of the need for compression and elevation of the left knee by the next treatment session.

The physical therapist also provided education about continuing to use the ace wrap for edema reduction and education about elevating the leg at night or when the patient was sitting. In addition, the physical therapist provided home exercises for strengthening the patient's right upper and lower extremities. These included:

1. Standing push-ups with the right upper extremity.
2. Horizontal abduction and adduction using a yellow theraband (minimal resistance).
3. Hip flexion in sitting, with instructions to keep her hands on the edge of the chair to minimize substitution.
4. Knee extension in sitting, using a red theraband (moderate resistance).

The physical therapist scheduled the patient to return in 1 week to evaluate progress and for any other potential problems related to mobility.

Intervention

TREATMENT SESSION ONE
Date: March 8

When the patient returned the next week, she reported pain in the neck and both shoulders. She believed it was related to using the walker. The physical therapist examined the patient's neck and both shoulders. The patient had muscle spasms in both upper trapezius muscles. She had pain with resisted shoulder flexion and adduction, as well as resisted shoulder shrugs. The patient rated her left arm pain as 7 out of 10, and her right shoulder pain as 6 out of 10.

How did the new symptoms change the plan of care? What recommendations could be made?

The physical therapist reviewed the patient's gait with the walker. Because of the weakness in her right side, the patient tended to use her left arm more to push the walker forward and to help support her right leg as she advanced her right leg. The patient had difficulty maintaining partial weight bearing of her left leg and again relied heavily on her left arm. The physical therapist surmised that her gait pattern with the walker was the cause of the shoulder and neck pain. Although the patient was using her left arm much more than her right, she was using her right arm more than she was used to, and thus had pain in both arms.

The physical therapist discussed the use of a scooter with the patient. The patient was opposed to the idea, stating that she was not ready to begin using a wheelchair or scooter. She said that she had worked very hard to be able to walk independently and was not ready to face using a chair again.

The physical therapist also discussed energy-conservation techniques with the patient. Recommendations included having the patient plan her day to minimize the amount of walking she needed to do, sitting for as many activities of daily living and instrumental activities of daily living as possible (e.g., grooming, showering, meal preparation), and considering the use of a delivery service for her groceries. The patient agreed to all of the recommendations except using a shower seat.

Because of the pain in the patient's right arm, the physical therapist told the patient to discontinue the right upper extremity strengthening exercises. The therapist reviewed her right lower extremity strengthening program and instructed her to continue with it. The therapist made an appointment for the patient to return in 2 weeks, after her next physician visit.

TREATMENT SESSION TWO
Date: March 22
At the next visit, the patient reported that she had attempted to walk without the walker, but that the pain and swelling in her knee had increased. She brought a new order from the physician for non–weight-bearing gait with the walker.

At her physician's visit, the patient reported that she had a second radiograph, which was still negative for fractures. The physician then ordered a bone scan, which showed possible heterotopic ossification (HO) in her left medial knee joint. The physician then decided on the non–weight-bearing gait order.

The patient reported that the pain in her shoulders and neck was worse. She reported constant fatigue related to increased energy costs of gait, and difficulty sleeping at night because of pain. She rated the pain in both arms as 10 out of 10. She also reported an increase in feelings of depression.

How did this new information change the plan of care? What new recommendations were necessary?

At this point, the physical therapist strongly recommended that the patient try a scooter. The therapist told the patient that the neck and shoulder pain was likely to decrease when she stopped using the walker. The physical therapist noted that because of difficulty maintaining a non–weight-bearing gait, the patient often returned to a partial weight-bearing gait. It was possible that this might be impeding healing. The physical therapist also reminded the patient that the use of the scooter was likely to be temporary, but that it could help prevent further HO and decrease the neck and shoulder pain. She also discussed the relationship between pain and depression. After the discussion, the patient agreed to try a scooter. The physical therapist arranged for the patient to meet with the local durable medical equipment supplier the following day.

The physical therapist also discussed the need for counseling with the patient, based on the patient's report of feelings of depression. The patient informed the physical therapist that she met regularly with a psychologist, with whom she had been discussing her current physical problems. The patient stated she was worried about how long she would be able to live in her current apartment, because she would be unable to get the scooter up the stairs. She also worried about how long she would be able to live independently if her physical status continued to decline.

What was an appropriate response to the patient's concerns?

The physical therapist encouraged the patient to discuss these issues with her psychologist. She also reminded the patient that the use of the scooter might be temporary and beneficial in promoting healing of the left leg. The physical therapist did encourage the patient to begin thinking about looking for a first-floor, accessible apartment. She pointed out the difficulties the patient had encountered with having to negotiate stairs with her current injury and also reminded her that it might be possible to use the scooter at home if she had a more accessible living situation.

At the end of the treatment session, the physical therapist and the patient reviewed the right lower extremity exercise program. The patient was able to perform all exercises without difficulty. The physical therapist added the following exercises:

- Mini-squats for the right leg, using the walker or a counter for support.
- Hip abduction in the side-lying position for both legs.

TREATMENT SESSION THREE
Date: March 23

The following day, the patient met with the durable medical equipment supplier and rented a scooter. The physical therapist reviewed the features of the scooter with the patient and assessed the patient's ability to negotiate the scooter and transfer in and out of it. The patient was independent in scooter mobility and transfers. Because of the inaccessibility of the patient's home, it was decided that the patient would use the scooter at work and use her walker at home. The physical therapist scheduled the patient for a follow-up visit in 1 week.

TREATMENT SESSION FOUR
Date: March 30

The patient reported that she had undergone a second bone scan and magnetic resonance imaging 2 days earlier. Both tests were positive for HO in the left medial knee. The patient was placed on indomethacin for 6 weeks to prevent further development of HO.

The physical therapist reviewed the patient's strengthening program. After consultation with the patient's physician, the physical therapist had the patient try using the exercise bike in the clinic. The patient was able to transfer on and off the bike independently and to tolerate riding the bike for 15 minutes at a moderate pace, with appropriate vital sign responses. The patient informed the physical therapist that she had a stationary bicycle in her apartment. The physical therapist recommended that the patient add riding the exercise bicycle for 15 to 20 minutes per day as part of her exercise program.

The physical therapist reviewed the patient's gait with the walker. Although her gait was slow, the patient was able to walk 100 feet and maintain non–weight-bearing with her left leg. It took her 6 minutes to walk 100 feet with the walker. During the 100 hundred feet, she took three breaks of 20 seconds each.

The patient reported no problems using the scooter. She stated that her back and neck pain had decreased steadily over the past week. Her left arm pain was now 4 out of 10 and her right arm pain was 3 out of 10. The physical therapist recommended that the patient resume the upper extremity exercises that were part of her original exercise program and advised her patient to discontinue the exercises if her pain level increased.

The physical therapist scheduled the patient to return in 1 week to review her gait and exercise program.

Reexamination
TREATMENT SESSION FIVE
Date: April 6

The patient reported that the pain in both upper extremities was unchanged from the week before. She felt that the continued pain was related to use of the walker. Examination of the patient's gait revealed that the patient demonstrated greater endurance while using the walker and was now able to walk 150 feet while maintaining her non–weight-bearing status. She was able to walk 100 feet with the walker in 4 minutes and did not take any rest breaks while walking.

The physical therapist reviewed the patient's exercise program. The patient was tolerating all of the exercises well, including the arm exercises that she had resumed the week earlier. The patient reported that she had ridden the stationary bicycle four times in the past week, for 15 minutes each time. Because of the length of the patient's current exercise program, the physical therapist decided not to add any new exercises at the time. The physical therapist made the following modifications:

- Use a red theraband (moderate resistance) for upper extremity exercises.
- Use a black theraband (maximal resistance) for lower extremity exercises.
- Attempt to increase the time on the stationary bicycle to 20 minutes per day, at least 4 days per week.

TREATMENT SESSION SIX

Date: April 13

The patient reported the pain in her left leg had decreased. She had new orders to begin partial weight-bearing gait with the walker, with progression to full weight-bearing as tolerated.

How could the patient's plan of care be changed given that she can bear weight on her left leg? Should she continue to use the scooter?

The therapist began with the patient performing some weight-shifting exercises while standing with the walker, and then progressed to gait with the walker. Compared with the initial examination, now the patient was able to shift her weight more smoothly onto her right side and to more easily shift weight between her left and right legs.

The physical therapist recommended that the patient continue to use the scooter at

work for long distances until her left leg was completely healed.

TREATMENT SESSIONS SEVEN TO TEN

Dates: April 20, 27, May 4, and May 11

The focus of treatment was now on improving gait with the walker and increasing tolerance to increased weight bearing on the left leg. Because of the patient's past history of back and neck pain related to her posture, the physical therapist and patient spent time working on the quality of gait. With practice, the patient was able to advance the right leg without circumducting it. The physical therapist worked with the patient on maintaining an equal step time and length on both legs, to help prevent her from reverting back to her old gait patterns.

New home exercises were as follows:

- Practice stepping on and off a stool without circumducting the right leg. The patient used her walker during the activity and needed to make sure that her right leg did not contact the walker as she was advancing it onto the stool.
- While standing in the walker, roll a ball back and forth with the left leg, for strength and balance training for the right leg.

In session nine, the patient began using her cane instead of the walker. The physical therapist worked with the patient to use the cane for balance instead of leaning on it heavily to support her weight. She reminded the patient that her right leg was stronger than it had been, and that she should need the cane less for support. During this session the physical therapist also began using the treadmill to help the patient work on weight shifting and stance time at varying speeds.

The patient and the physical therapist agreed that the patient could begin using her cane instead of the scooter for long distances. The physical therapist encouraged the patient to resume using the scooter if she experienced a return of knee, back, or neck pain.

Outcome and Discharge

TREATMENT SESSION ELEVEN: DISCHARGE

Date: May 18

The physical therapist repeated the tests and measures used during the initial examination.

Pain. The patient no longer had pain in the left knee or arms. She reported back pain as a 3 out of 10 after walking a long distance. She said the pain was relieved with rest.

Peripheral nerve integrity, muscle performance, and sensory integrity. *Sensation:* Intact throughout the left side. Sensation was decreased on the right side; the right leg was more affected than the right arm. Proprioception, kinesthesia, and sharp/dull testing were decreased in the right leg.

Strength: Because of the spasticity present on the right side, the physical therapist did not assign manual muscle test grades. The left arm and leg were functional throughout. The patient was able to elevate her right arm overhead 60 degrees. Elbow flexion was functional. She was able to fully extend her elbow in a gravity-eliminated position. She was able to extend her elbow 60 degrees against gravity. The patient had minimal motion in her right wrist and hand. Her wrist rested in neutral. Her hand rested in a clawed position. The patient was able to flex her right hip against gravity 50 degrees without using substitution. She was able to extend the right hip fully against gravity with moderate resistance. She was able to abduct her right hip when side-lying and standing 30 degrees. The patient was able to extend her right knee fully against gravity with moderate resistance. Increased resistance caused increased extensor tone throughout. The patient had minimal movement in ankle dorsiflexion and no active ankle plantarflexion.

Range of motion. The left side was functional throughout. The right shoulder exhibited decreased passive range of motion in shoulder elevation and external rotation. Wrist and fingers had limited motion in all planes. The right leg was functional except for ankle dorsiflexion and plantarflexion, which were both limited to 10 degrees.

Posture. The patient sat and stood with a slight posterior pelvic tilt, with more weight on the left side. The patient was able to achieve a neutral pelvis and equal weight-bearing on both legs with visual cues (e.g., a mirror). A slight forward head position was noted.

Gait, locomotion, and balance. The patient was using a single-point cane for all gait. Step length was nearly equal, with left step length slightly shorter than right. Occasional right hip hiking and circumduction were noted after patient had walked long distances.

The patient's Tinetti assessment tool score was 21/28, and her Berg balance scale score was 49/56. All goals established at the initial examination had been met.

The physical therapist instructed the patient to occasionally look in the mirror while walking to help correct right hip hiking and circumduction. She recommended that the patient continue with her home exercise program, especially riding the exercise bike and the exercises for lower extremity strengthening. The physical therapist told the patient that some of her improvements in gait might be due to the need for her right leg to support her weight while her left leg was healing. She described this as a form of constraint-induced movement therapy.

Finally, the physical therapist recommended that the patient come in for a reexamination in 4 to 6 weeks, to determine the need for further intervention to modify and improve her gait pattern.

RECOMMENDED READINGS

Berg K, Wood-Dauphinee S, Williams JI, Maki B: Measuring balance in the elderly: validation of an instrument, *Can J Public Health* 83(2):S7, 1992.

Blanton S, Wolf SL: An application of upper-extremity constraint-induced movement therapy in a patient with subacute stroke, *Phys Ther* 79:847, 1999.

Davies, PM: *Steps to follow: a guide to the treatment of adult hemiplegia*, New York: Springer-Verlag, 2000.

D'Lima DD, Venn-Watson EJ, Tripuraneni P, Colwell CW: Indomethacin versus radiation therapy for heterotopic ossification after hip arthroplasty, *Orthopedics* 24(12):1139, 2001.

American Physical Therapy Association: Guide to physical therapist practice, second edition, *Phys Ther* 81:1, 2001.

Fowler EG, Ho TW, Nwigwe AI, Dorey FJ: The effect of quadriceps femoris muscle strengthening exercises on spasticity in children with cerebral palsy, *Phys Ther* 81:1215, 2001.

Hertling D, Kessler RM, Kessler D, *Management of common musculoskeletal disorders: physical therapy principles and methods* (ed 3), Philadelphia: Lippincott Williams and Wilkins, 1996.

McKinley WO, Gittler MS, Kirshblum SC, et al: Spinal cord injury medicine. 2 medical complications after spinal cord injury: identification and management, *Arch Phys Med Rehabil* 83(3 Suppl 1):S58, S90, 2002.

O'Sullivan SB, Schmitz T: *Physical rehabilitation: assessment and treatment.* (ed 4), Philadelphia: FA Davis, 2001.

Sabari JS, Kane L, Flanagan SR, Steinberg A: Constraint-induced motor relearning after stroke: a naturalistic case report, *Arch Phys Med Rehabil* 82(4):524, 2001.

Shehab D, Elgazzar AH, Collier BD: Heterotopic ossification, *J Nucl Med* 43(3):346, 2002.

Stevenson TJ: Detecting change in patients with stroke using the Berg Balance Scale, *Aust J Physiother* 47(1):29, 2001.

Taub E, Uswatte G, Pidikiti R: Constraint-induced movement therapy: a new family of techniques with broad implication to physical rehabilitation—a clinical review, *J Rehabil Res Dev* 36(3):237, 1999.

Tinetti ME: Performance-oriented assessment of mobility problems in the elderly, *J Am Geriatr Soc* 34:119, 1986.

van der Lee JH, Beckerman H, Lankhorst GJ, Bouter LM: Constraint-induced movement therapy, *Phys Ther* 80(7):711, 2000.

Whitney SL, Poole JL, Cass SP: A review of balance instruments for older adults, *Am J Occup Ther* 52(8):666, 1998.

LEARNING OBJECTIVES

The reader will be able to:

1. Explain the importance of trunk strength and stability in infants and young children and its impact on all developmental areas.
2. Be able to develop treatment strategies that combine gross motor skill acquisition while concurrently impacting other areas (e.g., speech, fine motor skills).
3. Identify some clinical signs of trunk weakness.
4. Explain the importance of developing the trunk in three planes of movement.

Examination

HISTORY

The patient was a 22-month-old male with severe hypotonia and global developmental delay. He had been receiving physical therapy two times per week from an early intervention program in another county and was transferred to another facility when the family moved. The new physical therapist received a general overall evaluation from the previous physical therapist before the first session. On arriving at the house, the new therapist was able to obtain a brief history from the parents. The parents reported that the pregnancy and delivery were unremarkable. The patient had a history of infantile spasms beginning at age 3 weeks. At about 3 months, he was placed on adrenocorticotropic hormone therapy and Topomax to control the spasms. At the time of the initial visit, he was taking only Topomax, and no visible seizures were reported. He was being followed by a neurologist and an orthopedist. The family's primary physical therapy goal was for improved head control. Other goals included holding a toy for longer periods and continuing to work on making sounds.

TESTS AND MEASURES

After a brief physical examination, the physical therapist found passive range of motion to be within normal limits in all joints. When positioned supine, the child kept his head turned to the right and generally kept his extremities in abduction and external rotation. He was able to move them through a partial range of motion against gravity using small phasic bursts of movement. He was able to bring either hand to his mouth with his head turned to the side. He was unable to actively transition in or out of any position. When rolled over onto his stomach, he would right his head with his body. From the prone position, he was able to extend his head again using small bursts (with the head laterally tilted to the right) when given assistance to prop on his forearms. He was rounded forward into a kyphotic posture with head down into full flexion when held in long sitting. He required maximum assist to sit and keep his head up in midline. When the therapist attempted to hold him in supported standing, the therapist's hands slipped up his trunk, and the child was unable to take weight through his feet. It was difficult to obtain good alignment in any upright position.

Evaluation

Based on the examination results, intervention focused on teaching the family techniques to improve the patient's head, neck, and trunk control. This was done through activities with the patient in prone and supine positions on the floor and over a ball. It also included positioning while his mother was carrying him and positioning on the floor. Over the first 2 weeks of treatment, the therapist continued to evaluate the child's functional abilities, strengths, and needs.

During intervention, the patient would tire quickly and would complain if left on his belly too long on the floor or over a lap. When he cried or vocalized to complain, the duration was short. When he coughed, his entire body flexed forward in one burst and coughed no more than once each time. Further assessment of the child's breathing determined that he was primarily a diaphragmatic breather. In his rib cage, the ribs were flared and horizontally aligned with decreased intercostal spaces.

Diagnosis

Physical Therapist Practice Pattern 5B: Impaired Neuromotor Development.

Prognosis

GOALS

The patient will:

1. Move his head from left to right 180 degrees and back again while in prone and supine, in 1 year.
2. Maintain his head in an upright position for 30 seconds when placed in a position of supported prone on elbows, in 1 year.
3. Maintain chin tuck while reaching in supine or while assisted playing with his feet, in 1 year.

The prognosis for achieving these goals in 1 year is fair to good. Family interest and involvement is likely to drive achievement of these goals.

What would have been appropriate interventions at this point?

Intervention

After gathering the information from the brief history and evaluation, the therapist initially directed treatment toward improving head, neck, and trunk control. The patient did not have any independent movement in and out of positions and thus needed to begin to gain some proximal stability to begin to develop some overall muscular control.

The therapist began with activities to work on trunk strengthening in prone and supine and provided suggestions to the family for positioning. These activities were designed to work the child's abdominal muscles primarily in the sagittal plane. After further observation and assessment, the therapist determined that the internal and external obliques were not working actively. Importantly, the obliques needed to be addressed first, because of their effect on rib cage development and thus on trunk mobility and breathing.

Contraction of the obliques creates a downward pull at the bottom of the ribs, changing their shape and alignment. This downward movement increases the size of the rib space, allowing the intercostal muscles to be more active. The obliques work with the intercostals and rectus abdominus to anchor the rib cage and help create a pressure gradient so that the diaphragm, the primary respiratory muscle, can work efficiently.

Using this knowledge, the therapist altered the plan of care to focus more on strengthening all of the abdominal muscles in all three planes of movement. Such treatment strategies as downward vibration through the rib cage, rolling, playing while side-lying, and playing with feet were added. Positioning strategies were also adjusted using towel rolls and pillows to improve alignment and to help open up his intercostal spaces.

In the weeks that followed, the family began to express their frustration with the child's global developmental delay and his slow progress. His mother stated that she would like to try feeding him more textured foods, like cereal, in addition to the pureed baby food that he was eating. She also said that she wanted her son to be able to hold his bottle by himself, because as he was getting bigger it was progressively becoming more difficult to feed him on her lap. She requested these goals be added to the physical therapy plan of care.

What interventions would have been appropriate?

The physical therapist obtained consultations from a speech therapist and an occupational therapist so that a more comprehensive treatment plan could be implemented. The speech therapist recommended initiating therapy once weekly to address the feeding concerns and provided the family with suggestions for activities for oral stimulation and exploration. The occupational therapist provided suggestions for increasing sensory input and awareness.

They decided to begin sessions with a lotion massage to increase the child's body awareness by providing tactile input. In addition, they decided to incorporate more movement in various directions with the child on the ball, to increase vestibular input. The vestibular system assists in head control and helps keep the head upright so the eyes are at a horizontal level. Movement through different planes is meant to give the child varied movement experiences that he is unable to give himself.

After the sensory preparation, the therapists worked with the child side-lying on helping him hold a teether and bring it to his mouth to provide oral stimulation. This position helped the child bring both hands together in midline while eliminating gravity.

The physical therapist also talked to the family about their questions regarding feeding and holding a bottle. They discussed normal development and the development of muscular strength. They talked about how a child needs to develop a point of stability from which skills can be built and that the trunk is the point of stability from which the head and the extremities work. A lack of stability proximally makes it much more difficult to develop refined skills in distal areas, such as the arms and hands to hold a bottle, and the mouth to chew and swallow textured foods.

The physical therapist and family collaborated on determining safe positions for feeding the child. The optimal position included providing maximal proximal support while bringing the child out of his preferred postures into capital flexion (chin tuck), bringing his shoulders back into thoracic extension, and maintaining a midline symmetrical posture.

The mother and child had difficulty with the change, and so two options were developed to help them adjust. The first option was a semireclining seat with rolled towels placed around the child's head and neck to keep them in midline and out of hyperextension and additional towels on each side of his trunk to keep the spine aligned. The second option included progression to an adapted seat in a semireclining position with head and trunk supports. This proved the best option for overall alignment. The mother began putting the child in the adapted seat for a small snack during the day and progressed from one meal to three, and from a semi-reclining position to a more upright one.

Outcome

Therapy continued over the next year with carryover at home through the family's daily activities including bath, play, and mealtimes. Formal reexaminations were performed every 6 months. The child began to develop increased head and trunk control (e.g., to maintain head/neck extension in a prone position on elbows), and interventions were modified to reduce external supports. An example of these modifications was to reduce the number of towel rolls used to support the upper extremities and trunk.

Within the year, attention also began to focus on the child's transition to school when he turned 3 years old. The family and therapist worked together on seating and transportation issues as his birthday approached. At the appropriate time, the child entered an adapted preschool program.

Discussion

When treating children under age 3 years, the physical therapist must remember that all areas of development are interrelated. In this particular case, the development of gross motor skills was delayed because of the child's global hypotonia. This overall weakness led to delays in all developmental areas stemming from trunk weakness severe enough to prohibit the child from moving independently. The child's lack of independent movement prevented him from exploring his body and environment, further affecting development of gross motor skills as well as cognition, fine motor skills, self-feeding, and language.

The trunk plays an important role in this development, providing a point of stability from which the head and extremities work. When the base is unstable, distal control is subsequently compensated for, which affects how well the child can use his hands, feet, mouth, eyes, and other structures.

A child should be assessed in various positions, including prone, supine, and upright postures, enabling the therapist to evaluate the child's ability to move against gravity. Physical and audible clues, such as duration and loudness of vocalizations, changes in vocalizations and respirations with changes in posture, quality of cough, and breathholding during movement, should be noted. Further physical assessment of breathing and the rib cage—including evaluation of rib cage size, shape, and symmetry; alignment and spacing of ribs; breathing pattern; and spinal alignment—was important in this case.

The results of the assessment were used in correlation with knowledge of normal development to devise a more comprehensive treatment plan. Consultations from other disciplines can also help ensure incorporation of all developmental areas into treatment strategies therefore optimizing interventions and the child's learning.

RECOMMENDED READINGS

Stamer M: *Posture and movement of the child with cerebral palsy*, San Antonio, Texas: Therapy Skill Builders, 2000.

Tecklin JS (ed): *Pediatric physical therapy* (ed 3), Philadelphia: Lippincott, 2000.

LEARNING OBJECTIVES

The reader will be able to:

1. Correlate the patient's symptoms with objective clinical findings.
2. Identify an appropriate physical therapy diagnosis and outline a plan of care in a case with multiple areas of involvement.

The reader should know that the patient was a 33-year-old male store manager who presented with complaints of low back pain with left anterior hip and thigh symptoms. He also reported symptoms that extended along the course of his right lateral thigh and leg. He stated that his symptoms began gradually approximately 18 months earlier. His symptoms were intermittent in nature and aggravated with bending, lifting, and prolonged sitting. In addition, prolonged standing and walking both produced and worsened his complaints. His symptoms were less in the morning and worse as his day progressed. He had a history of two prior episodes of acute lumbar pain during the previous 8 years. Each previous episode resolved spontaneously without formal intervention 3 to 5 days after onset. The patient spent most of his workday standing or walking, interspersed with periods of time at his desk. His general health was unremarkable. He enjoyed an active lifestyle, including aerobic conditioning and various sporting activities. Imaging studies included lumbar radiographs that suggested mild degenerative joint disease throughout the L3-4, L4-5, and L5-S1 levels. He had been referred to physical therapy with a diagnosis of low back pain.

Based on the patient's reports of aggravating activities, what structures were being stressed?

Examination

Based on the patient's history, symptomatology, and subjective reports of aggravating activities, the examination focused on screening procedures for both the lumbar spine and hips. The patient's standing posture demonstrated a normal lumbar lordosis with no apparent asymmetries. His sitting posture was poor, characterized by a moderately flexed lumbar spine, protracted shoulders, and forward head. Examination revealed active range of motion (ROM) of his lumbar spine that was mildly restricted in flexion and moderately restricted in extension. Lateral bending and rotation ROM appeared to be within normal limits. Lower extremity dermatome, myotome, and reflex scans each appeared within normal limits. Neural tension signs were negative for the sciatic nerve. Repeated motion testing of the lumbar spine produced and worsened right lumbar, lateral thigh, and leg pain with flexion of the lumbar spine in standing. Lumbar spine extension in standing decreased and abolished his right lumbar, lateral thigh, and leg symptoms. Passive ROM of his left hip revealed marked restrictions in both internal rotation and abduction. Passive hip flexion and extension were each moderately restricted, whereas external rotation was mildly restricted on the left side.[1] Resisted isometrics of the left hip were strong and painless for each of the major muscle groups. The patient's free speed gait pattern was characterized by a lack of left hip extension from midstance to preswing (toe-off).

Evaluation

The patient was demonstrating lumbar pain that extended over the course of his right L5 dermatome that was produced with repeated or sustained lumbar flexion. He also demonstrated a lack of lumbar extension ROM. A restriction of left hip passive ROM in a capsular pattern was present. Gait deviations consistent with a lack of passive left hip extension ROM were also noted.

How does limited hip ROM influence function of the lumbar spine?

A lack of passive hip flexion ROM places greater ROM demands on the lumbar spine and pelvis and consequently increases lumbar stress when the patient is required to forward flex the lumbar spine and hips from either the sitting or standing positions. The same is true when extending the lumbar spine in standing when a lack of passive hip extension ROM is present. Dysfunction at one joint can often lead to compensatory dysfunction at an adjacent joint.

Diagnosis

Physical Therapist Practice Patterns 4F: Impaired Joint Mobility, Motor Function, Muscle Performance, Range of Motion and Reflex Integrity Associated with Spinal Disorders and 4D: Impaired Joint Mobility, Motor Function, Muscle Performance, Range of Motion Associated with Capsular Restriction.

Prognosis

GOALS

The patient will:
1. Exhibit restoration of full lumbar extension ROM and abolished right lower extremity referred symptoms in 3 weeks.
2. Demonstrate improved passive ROM of the left hip to mild restrictions with internal rotation and abduction, with full restoration of hip flexion and extension passive ROM in 8 weeks.
3. Resolve associated left lower extremity referred symptoms in 8 weeks.
4. Normalize free-speed gait pattern as hip extension ROM is restored.

Intervention

The patient's lumbar symptoms were addressed using therapeutic exercises based on McKenzie

principles for lumbar derangement including extension in prone lying, which was performed every waking 2 hours.[2] The patient was also encouraged to avoid periods in high-stress spinal postures, particularly prolonged sitting and bending from the waist. A lumbar roll was issued for use during the times when he was required to sit. His left hip capsular restriction was addressed with stretching exercises for hip abduction, internal rotation, flexion, and extension to be performed for a minimum of 2 minutes in each direction, four times per day.

Outcome

The patient was reexamined at 3 weeks, at which time he demonstrated full lumbar extension and a complete resolution of his lumbar and right lower extremity referred symptoms. However, he continued to experience significant restrictions in his left hip ROM and the onset of left anterior hip and thigh symptoms after extended periods of weight bearing. The patient was referred back to his primary care physician because of a lack of meaningful progress with his left hip condition. His primary care physician in turn ordered further imaging studies. A radiograph of his left hip suggested end-stage degenerative changes. Subsequent magnetic resonance imaging suggested femoral head avascular necrosis. The patient continued to perform his left hip stretching exercises on a home basis before undergoing a cementless total hip arthroplasty 24 months later.[3]

REFERENCES

1. Hertling D, Kessler R: *Management of common musculoskeletal disorders: physical therapy principles and methods* (ed 3), Philadelphia: Lippincott, 1996.
2. McKenzie RA: *The lumbar spine: mechanical diagnosis and therapy*, Waikanae, New Zealand: Spinal Publications, 1981.
3. Hellman EJ, Capello WN, Feinberg JR: Omnifit cementless total hip arthroplasty: a 10-year average followup, *Clin Orthop* 364:164, 1999.

LEARNING OBJECTIVES

The reader will be able to:

1. Describe the pathophysiology of psoriasis.
2. Differentiate psoriatic arthritis from other joint dysfunctions.
3. Display knowledge of the psychosocial issues associated with psoriasis.
4. Recognize common impairments and functional limitations of a person with psoriasis.
5. Identify pertinent examination and evaluation elements for a person with psoriasis.
6. Describe the benefits of phototherapy and photochemotherapy interventions in the treatment of psoriasis.
7. Identify risk factors of phototherapy and photochemotherapy.
8. State specific phototherapy goals for this patient.

The reader should know that the patient was a 38-year-old white male with ongoing psoriasis. He worked as an accountant at a local firm. He began seeing scattered spots of psoriasis when he was 19 or 20 years old. In the past 10 to 12 years, his psoriasis became progressively worse. He reported that, from increased job-related stresses and at certain times of the year, his psoriasis would flare up.

What are the etiology, incidence, risk factors, pathogenesis, clinical manifestations, and prognosis of psoriasis?

Psoriasis is a noncontagious, chronic, inflammatory dermatosis characterized by elevated erythematous plaques covered with dry, silvery scales. Its cause is unknown. Heredity contributes to development of psoriasis in about one third of the cases, but the role of genetic factors is not clear. Current research indicates that there is an immune-mediated dysfunction in families with psoriasis. The normal life cycle of a skin cell is 28 days; however, the turnover time of psoriatic skin is 3 to 4 days. Psoriasis is represented equally in both genders and is most common in young adults, with a mean onset at age 27. It affects about 1% to 2% of Caucasians and is uncommon in African-Americans. Flare-ups are unpredictable, but may be related to systemic and/or environmental factors. Trauma, infection (especially hemolytic streptococci), pregnancy, and endocrinologic changes are frequent precipitating systemic factors. Cold weather and emotional stress or severe anxiety may also exacerbate psoriasis. Psoriasis can be physically disfiguring and emotionally disabling, and can have a distressing effect on the lives of both the individual and his or her family.[1-6]

Examination and Evaluation

The patient's most recent flare-up of psoriasis followed a severe strep throat infection. When the patient presented to the dermatologist, he had 55% to 65% body coverage of moderately thick plaques that were thicker and larger on his knees and elbows. Occasional plaques on the palmar surfaces of his hands and plantar surfaces of his feet were painful and limited his ability to perform some activities of daily living. Ambulation for more than short distances was also difficult. The dermatologist confirmed the diagnosis of psoriasis with a punch skin biopsy and prescribed several increasingly stronger topical corticosteroids.

The patient saw the dermatologist every 3 to 4 weeks for 6 months, but despite this medical intervention, his psoriasis became progressively worse. He also received two courses of antibiotic therapy during that time secondary to topical skin infections. The dermatologist decided to try phototherapy and referred the patient to the light therapy center in the physical therapy department at his local hospital.

How should a person with psoriasis be examined and evaluated?

Elements of examination and evaluation include history of previous skin treatment, including topical applications, light therapy, photosensitizing medication, and radiation therapy. Initial skin assessment includes skin typing, description of extent and type of skin lesion, duration, factors causing flares and remissions, itching, history of "cold sores," observation of skin scalp and nails, and identification of any other discomforts. A body diagram is helpful for documenting the extent of lesions and progression of healing. Additional essential data to collect include concomitant medical problems, family history of skin disease, and any other medications that the patient may be taking. Several common medications, including tetracycline, thiazide diuretics, and oral contraceptives, can increase photosensitivity.[7]

The patient's general health was good, and he had few other medical problems. His father had severe psoriasis, and his grandfather had a skin disorder of unknown origin. The patient exercised two to three times per week and was involved in occasional social activities. However, he usually avoided outdoor activities where he might need to wear short-sleeved shirts or shorts. He enjoyed playing golf, but played only during the early spring or late fall when the temperatures were cool enough that he could comfortably wear a long-sleeved jersey and long pants.

The patient had never received any type of phototherapy or radiation therapy, and he was not taking any medications. Through his self-reported erythema and pigment response to natural sunlight, he was classified as skin type II (always burns, sometimes tans). A body diagram was completed, noting the type and extent of his skin lesions (Figure 30-1). His range of motion, muscle strength, and sensa-

tion were all within normal limits at the time of the examination. He was given a *minimal erythema dose* (MED) test on his arm to determine his sensitivity to ultraviolet light. (The MED is the smallest dose of ultraviolet radiation that yields erythema that is just detectable by eye after 8 to 24 hours of exposure.) Individuals may also be classified according to their self-reported erythema and pigmentary response to natural sunlight exposure.[7,8]

Diagnosis

Physical Therapy Practice Pattern 7C: Impaired Integumentary Integrity Associated with Partial-Thickness Skin Involvement and Scar Formation.

Prognosis

At the end of the plan of care, the patient was expected to have 80% to 90% clearing of his disease. The dermatologist and physical therapist had biweekly meetings in which the amount and extent of disease was diagrammed and reviewed to reassess and determine the best course of therapeutic intervention for the patient.

Intervention

The patient was taught about the etiology of psoriasis and how ultraviolet radiation slows the overproduction of skin cells and mildly strengthens the immune system. Phototherapy or ultraviolet B light band (UVB) therapy was initiated at 20% below the patient's MED, or at 35 mjoules. (Broad-band UVB has been an accepted treatment for psoriasis for decades and works for about two thirds of patients. UVB is considered when topical treatments, such as ointments and corticosteroids, are not effective.) The UVB dose was increased by 20% to 30% per treatment as tolerated. The patient was seen three times a week for 6 weeks. He was reevaluated at the beginning of each session and asked to report his erythema at approximately 6 to 8 hours after the session. This information was then used to determine the next UVB dose.

LIGHT THERAPY CENTER ASSESSMENT

Previous Patient: _____

Name: _____

Age: _____

Address: _____

_____

Insurance: _____

Daytime Phone #: _____

Occupation: _____

Date: _____ Time: _____

Physician: _____

Diagnosis: _____

_____

Add'l Med. Problems: _____

Medications: _____

_____

Previous Light Rx: _____

_____

Previous Skin Treatment:

    Topical:

    Light Therapy:

    Photosensitizing Meds:

    Radiation Therapy:

Skin Assessment at First Treatment:

Subjective:

    Skin Type:

    Extent:

    Duration:

    Factors Causing:

        Flare

        Remission

    Itching:

    Discomfort:

    History of "Cold Sores":

Objective:

    Lesion Type:

    Hair/Scalp:

    Nails:

Goal of Therapy:　　Clearance of Skin Disease

Family History of Skin Disease: _____

_____

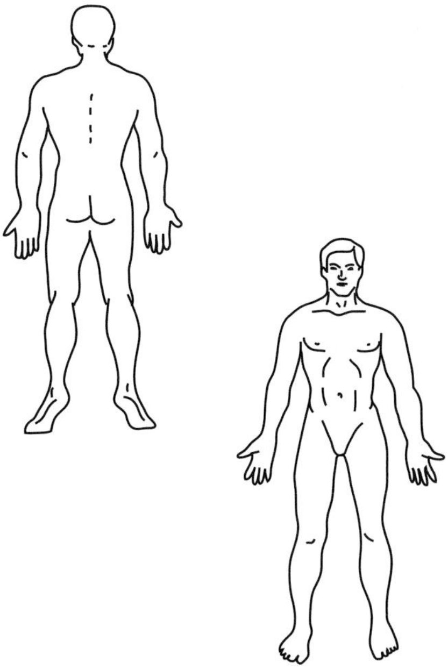

Therapist:

FIGURE 30-1 Sample body diagram (©Michael B. Ashley, PT, Ashley & Kuzma Physical Therapy and Photomedicine, Erie, Penn. Used with permission.)

Continued

Light Therapy Review	Rx #:	Date:
Response:		Physical Findings:
Compliance:		
Complications:		
UVA/UVB Dosage:		
Medications:		
Clearing/Maint.	Rx/wk:	
Changes:		
Reviewer:		

Light Therapy Review	Rx #:	Date:
Response:		Physical Findings:
Compliance:		
Complications:		
UVA/UVB Dosage:		
Medications:		
Clearing/Maint.	Rx/wk:	
Changes:		
Reviewer:		

Light Therapy Review	Rx #:	Date:
Response:		Physical Findings:
Compliance:		
Complications:		
UVA/UVB Dosage:		
Medications:		
Clearing/Maint.	Rx/wk:	
Changes:		
Reviewer:		

Addressograph	Monthly Phototherapy Progress Notes

FIGURE 30-1, cont'd For legend see p. 137.

Three weeks after beginning phototherapy, the patient reported increased pain in his right elbow and hands after a weekend during which he played three rounds of golf, because the weather was finally comfortable enough for him to wear long sleeves and pants.

What are the incidence, etiology, and clinical manifestations of psoriatic arthritis?

The possibility of psoriatic arthritis should be considered for all persons known to have psoriasis and exhibit any type of joint dysfunction. Approximately 10% to 30% of persons with psoriasis develop psoriatic arthritis. It commonly affects one or more joints of the fingers or toes and has a predilection for the distal interphalangeal joints of the hands. There may be nail changes including separation from the nail bed and/or pitting that mimics fungal infections. Usually, psoriatic arthritis tends to develop slowly, with mild symptoms and less joint tenderness, leading to misdiagnosis and/or underestimation of its severity.[5,6]

Reexamination

The pain in the patient's elbow resolved in 3 to 4 days, but it took about 10 days for the pain in his hands to go away. Because this appeared to be an isolated and justifiable incident of joint pain, the dermatologist and physical therapist decided to just monitor his joints.

The patient tolerated phototherapy well and had very few episodes of pinkness or soreness. Generally, he was increased 20% to 30% per treatment up to a dose of 450 mjoules. However, after 15 treatments, the patient demonstrated only a fair response, or about a 30% reduction in plaques. It was determined that the broad-band UVB was not as effective for this patient, and after consultation with the dermatologist, PUVA therapy (consisting of psoralen, an oral medication drug that increases photosensitivity, and ultraviolet A light band [UVA] phototherapy) was recommended. PUVA is typically considered for persons who have moderate to severe psoriasis and who have been resistant to other types of treatments.[2,8,9]

What risk factors and safeguards are associated with UVB and PUVA treatment interventions?

The main side effect of UVB is severe erythema causing blistering and subsequent peeling of skin. Despite the fact that sun exposure is a major risk factor in the development of skin cancer, no additional risk from UVB phototherapy has been reported.

Although PUVA treatments have been associated with an increased risk of skin cancer (particularly of nonaggressive forms, such as squamous cell and basal cell carcinoma), this risk has also been shown to be dose dependent.[2,8] Stern et al[10] reported a slightly increased risk of melanoma skin cancer in patients who had undergone long-term, high-dose PUVA (11 cases in 1380 subjects followed for 21 years). Current PUVA risks are minimized through sophisticated measuring devices and protection of sensitive areas (e.g., wearing protective eyeglasses for 12 to 24 hours, applying sunscreen to uninvolved areas, shielding male genitalia, and avoiding sunlight for 24 hours after ingesting psoralen).[2]

Intervention

The patient was taught about PUVA therapy and how to protect his skin and eyes while taking photosensitizing medications. The patient was advised to put on sunglasses and apply a sunscreen immediately after swallowing his medication. Between 1½ and 2 hours after receiving his oral medication of 30 mg of oxsralen-ultra (a psoralen-type drug), he received 1.0 joule of UVA; this amount was increased by 0.5 joule each treatment session per protocol. (Note that the UVB phototherapy standard of administration is in mjoules and that of UVA is in joules.) A new body diagram was made. At the beginning of each subsequent treatment session, the patient was reexamined and asked to report any erythema he may have experienced approximately 24 to 48 hours after the last treatment session. He was scheduled three times a week for treatment, and provided that he did turn pink or report soreness, his dosage was increased according to protocol.

Outcome

After nine treatments, the patient was showing clinical clearing of disease. At the twenty-fourth treatment, he had significant (90%+) clearing of disease, with only mild discoloration on his trunk and lower legs and a few thin spots on his elbows. Extra exposure on arms and legs was instituted by having the patient wear a gown for part of the treatment so that those areas could be exposed to UVA longer. By the twenty-sixth treatment, the patient was completely clear. After discussion with the dermatologist, he was placed on a weaning program two times per week for 2 weeks and then once a week for 2 weeks. Eventually he was tapered down to once per month. He was then discharged from photochemotherapy and monitored by his dermatologist.

After several months, the patient began having recurrences, indicating the need for a long-term maintenance program for his psoriasis. It was decided that the patient would obtain a home UVB unit. The physical therapist helped him obtain approval from the insurance company and a UVB unit delivered. The physical therapist made a home visit to calibrate the unit and instruct the patient in its use. After the home visit, the patient was monitored through several telephone calls to make sure he understood how to use it and was safely tolerating it. The patient now treats himself once every 10 to 14 days with a very small dose of UVB light and has been keeping his skin clear of psoriasis without the use of topical corticosteroids or oral medications. Currently, his skin has been clear for 8 months. He will continue with this regimen. During the summer, he will take a break from his phototherapy to get more natural sunlight exposure. He now enjoys playing golf throughout the summer.

Discussion

The patient in this case study needs to continue phototherapy treatments through the fall and winter, treating his skin every 7 to 10 days to keep the psoriasis under control. His long-term prognosis is that he will more than likely have a flare-up every 6 to 18 months that may require more aggressive treatment at times. The nature of psoriasis is highly individualized and unpredictable, because it is closely linked to the immune system. There is no known cure for psoriasis, only control measures to treat it.[1-3]

REFERENCES

1. Goodman CC, Boissonnault WG: *Pathology: implications for the physical therapist,* Philadelphia: WB Saunders, 1998.
2. National Psoriasis Foundation: *PUVA,* Portland, Oregon: National Psoriasis Foundation, 1999.
3. Psoriasis. In *Miller-Keane encyclopedic dictionary of medicine, nursing and allied health,* Philadelphia: WB Saunders, 1997.
4. National Psoriasis Foundation: *Psoriasis: questions and answers,* Portland, Oregon: National Psoriasis Foundation, 2000.
5. Goodman CC, Boissonnault WG: *Pathology: implications for the physical therapist,* Philadelphia: WB Saunders, 1998.
6. National Psoriasis Foundation: *Psoriatic arthritis,* Portland, Oregon: National Psoriasis Foundation, 1999.
7. Davis JM: Ultraviolet therapy. In Prentice WE (ed): *Therapeutic modalities for physical therapists,* New York: McGraw-Hill, 2002.
8. Diffey B, Farr P: Ultraviolet therapy. In Kitchen S, Bazin S (eds): *Electrotherapy: evidence-based practice,* Philadelphia: Churchill Livingstone, 2001.
9. Shelk J, Morgan P: Narrow-band UVB: a practical approach, *Dermatol Nurs* 12:407, 2000.
10. Stern RS, Nichols KT, Vakeva LH: Malignant melanoma in patients treated for psoriasis with methoxalen (psoralen) and ultraviolet B radiation (PUVA), *New Engl J Med* 336:1041, 1997.

RESOURCE

Persons with psoriasis, their families, and friends founded and continue to direct the National Psoriasis Foundation. They are committed through education, advocacy, and research to improve the quality of life for people who have psoriasis. They welcome requests for information and are a past recipient of the American Academy of Dermatology's Excellence in Education Award.

National Psoriasis Foundation
6600 SW 92nd Avenue, Suite 300
Portland OR 97223-7195
800-723-9166 or 503-244-7404
Fax: 503-245-0626
E-mail: getinfo@npfusa.org
Website: www.psoriasis.org

LEARNING OBJECTIVES

The reader will be able to:

1. Describe the signs and symptoms of chronic obstructive pulmonary disease (COPD).
2. Describe how the disease affects the functional capacity and quality of life of an individual with COPD.
3. Explain how to accurately and safely prescribe activity levels for patients with COPD.
4. Determine the appropriate use of oxygen therapy for the patient with COPD.

Examination

HISTORY

The patient was a 65-year-old retired bus driver. He had been married for 42 years, and had a 66-pack-year history of cigarette smoking. His wife encouraged him to stop smoking ever since she had quit 13 years ago after sustaining a myocardial infarction. The couple has two grown children and three grandchildren, but they do not visit very often because "grandpa" quickly becomes short of breath and tires easily. After years of progressively worsening bouts of shortness of breath, he was diagnosed with emphysema at age 59. Shortly after the COPD diagnosis was made, he was forced to take early retirement. He continued to be socially active in his community, however.

What signs and symptoms would be typical for a patient with emphysema?

Chest radiographs done at the time revealed hyperinflated lungs, flattened diaphragm, and a moderately enlarged heart. Subsequent testing demonstrated a slow, but continuous progression of the disease process. During the past year, the patient was hospitalized several times for acute respiratory infections. Three months ago he was hospitalized for 2 weeks with severe chest pain, which turned out to be pneumococcal pneumonia and pleurisy. During that hospital stay, the patient was placed on antibiotics and received chest physical therapy and respiratory therapy. The pneumonia left him very weak, with a dramatically decreased functional capacity to perform activities of daily living (ADL). His physician referred him to physical therapy as an outpatient in the pulmonary rehabilitation program.

SYSTEMS REVIEW

The patient had no significant neurologic or integumentary system findings, and his orthopedic examination was unremarkable except for muscle weakness of the lower extremities. He averaged a strength grade of 3/5 for the major muscle groups of the upper and lower extremities. His other signs and symptoms were limited to the pulmonary and cardiovascular systems.

The patient's predicted maximal oxygen capacity, based on gender, age, and activity level, was 28.8 mL/kg/minute (or 8.2 metabolic equivalents [METS]). (1 MET = 3.5 L oxygen/kg of body weight.) He attained a level of 10.5 mL/kg/minute (3 METS) on a graded exercise stress test using the Balke-Ware protocol. Therefore, he had a functional aerobic impairment (FAI) of 63.5%, which is considered marked impairment of aerobic capacity. (FAI = predicted maximal oxygen consumption – observed maximal oxygen consumption/predicted oxygen consumption × 100.)

Arterial blood gas (ABG) values are listed in Table 31-1, and pulmonary function test (PFT) values are given in Table 31-2.

TABLE 31-1
ARTERIAL BLOOD GAS VALUES

OBSERVED VALUES	NORMAL
pH 7.33	7.35-7.45
$PaCO_2$ 46 mm Hg	35-45 mm Hg
PaO_2 58 mm Hg	>80 mm Hg
HCO_3 29 mEq/L	22-28 mEq/L
O_2 Sat 88%	>90%

TABLE 31-2
PULMONARY FUNCTION TEST DATA

PULMONARY FUNCTION TEST	OBSERVED	PREDICTED
FEV_1	78%	>90%
FVC	2.75 L	4.11 L
FEV_1/FVC (%)	46%	70%
TLC	7.00 L	6.98 L

How could the 6-minute walk have been used to assess the patient's functional capacity?

The patient performed the 6-minute walk and was able to cover 320 meters, but had to stop several times due to dyspnea. At rest he reported a dyspnea level of 2/4, but while walking, his dyspnea level rose to 3/4, and it reached 4/4 when he was forced to stop and rest. (The dyspnea scale is as follows: 1, mild, noticeable to patient, not to observer; 2, some difficulty, noticeable to observer; 3, moderate difficulty, but can continue; 4, severe difficulty cannot continue.)

His oxygen saturation level, as measured by pulse oximetry, was 88% at rest, and it dropped to as low as 82% during portions of the 6-minute walk.

Diagnosis

Physical Therapist Practice Pattern 6C: Impaired Ventilation, Respiration/Gas Exchange, and Aerobic Capacity/Endurance Associated with Airway Clearance Dysfunction.

Prognosis

GOALS

All of the following goals were expected to be accomplished during a 12-week pulmonary rehabilitation program in which the patient exercised three to five times per week for 30 to 45 minutes per session:

1. Improve aerobic capacity to 14.0 mL/kg/minute (4 METS).
2. Improve muscle strength so that he is at a MMT grade of at least 4/5 in all the major muscle groups of the upper and lower extremities and the trunk.
3. Improve the ABG profile so that resting $PaCO_2$ level drops within the normal range of 35 to 45 mm Hg and PaO_2 improves to at least 70 mm Hg, as measured with a pulse oximeter.
4. Reduce smoking and stop completely by the end of the 12-week pulmonary rehabilitation program.
5. Avoid recurrence of acute respiratory infection for 1 year.

EXPECTED OUTCOME

All of the expected outcomes will be attained by the end of the 12-week pulmonary rehabilitation program:

1. The patient's 6-minute walk distance will increase without decreasing his oxygen saturation and increasing his RPE and perception of dyspnea.
2. The patient will perform ADL and self-care activities with less dyspnea.
3. The patient will increase to a level of 4/5 or greater for the major muscle groups of the upper and lower extremities.
4. The patient's increased mobility and pulmonary function will result in fewer respiratory infections.
5. The patient will stop smoking cigarettes.

Intervention

What is the benefit of long-term oxygen therapy for COPD patients?

It was determined that long-term (at least 19 hours per day) oxygen therapy was indicated. Long-term oxygen therapy has been shown to improve the quality of life for COPD patients by improving their psychological outlook, enhancing exercise performance, and improving skeletal-muscle metabolism. Long-term oxygen therapy is the only treatment known to increase the longevity of individuals with COPD.

Why was selecting the correct oxygen delivery device important?

An oxygen concentrator capable of filling portable containers was the device of choice, because it would provide the patient with an economical oxygen source at home, allow him to move about and remain socially active, and perform his ADL. Because Medicare paid for one device, it was important that the most appropriate device for this particular patient be selected. A pulse oximeter was also purchased so that the patient could monitor his oxygen saturation level and adjust the oxygen flow rate in response to his activity levels.

What were some areas of patient education appropriate for this patient?

The patient completed a 12-week pulmonary rehabilitation program. A significant portion of the program was dedicated to patient and family education. He was taught to monitor his own pulse rate, perception of dyspnea, and rate of perceived exertion (RPE). In addition, he and his wife were instructed in the use of the oxygen concentrator and pulse oximeter.

During the stress test, the patient was able to perform at a level of 3 METs, or 10.5 mL/kg/minute at a heart rate of 144 beats per minute before stopping the test because of dyspnea.

The physical therapist developed an exercise prescription with an intensity, duration, and frequency appropriate for the patient's condition and current functional status. The patient combined the stationary bicycle with a walking program, exercised 3 days a week at the clinic, and continued the walking program at home on his off days. The therapist taught him the proper way to warm up and cool down, breathing exercises, and a low-intensity weight-training program. The patient enjoyed relaxation training and attended smoking cessation classes.

Discharge Plan

The patient was discharged from pulmonary rehabilitation when he was able to perform ADL and self-care activities at a level of 3 to 4 METs using his oxygen delivery system and oximeter at a dyspnea level no greater than 2/4.

What are some activities within the patient's MET range?

MET values for some common activities are as follows:
- Eating 1.5
- Dressing 2.5
- Bathing 2.0
- Showering 4.0
- Driving car 2.0
- Light play with children 2.5 to 2.8
- Pumping gasoline 2.5
- Light housecleaning 2.5 to 3.5
- Fishing (sitting in boat) 2.5

Outcome

The patient was able to walk 440 meters (an increase of 25%) in 6 minutes with several rests and only mild dyspnea. His ABG and PFT profiles improved slightly (Tables 31-3 and 31-4). His muscle strength increased to an average of 4/5 in the major muscle groups of the extremities. He could not stop smoking completely, but was able to cut down from 1½ packs a day to ½ pack a day and continued to attend the smoking cessation program in hopes of completely quitting.

The patient was able to properly use his oxygen delivery and monitoring system. His maximal oxygen consumption increased to 13.5 mL/kg/min (3.86 METS), which decreased his FAI to 53% and classified his impairment as moderate rather than marked.

Discussion

Emphysema is a progressive disease that cannot be cured. However, with proper management,

TABLE 31-3
ARTERIAL BLOOD GAS VALUES
FOLLOWING INTERVENTION

ARTERIAL BLOOD GAS VALUES
pH 7.37
P_2CO_2 42 mm Hg
P_2O_2 60 mm Hg
HCO_3 28 mEq/L
O_2 Sat 92%

TABLE 31-4
PULMONARY FUNCTION TEST
FOLLOWING INTERVENTION

	OBSERVED
FEV_1	80%
FVC	2.76L
FEV_1/FVC (%)	46%
TLC	7.05 L

an individual can improve his or her quality of life despite the disease. Without proper management, an affected individual's quality of life and longevity will rapidly deteriorate. What is the most important thing this patient can do to manage his disease? Stopping smoking would do more to help this patient than any other intervention.

Patient education is very important, because there are many misconceptions about COPD. Exercise, done properly, helped this patient. But exercise done improperly could have made him more dyspneic, anxious, and frus-trated in his effort to improve his physical condition. Finally, educating the COPD patient on the use of oxygen is essential. The oxygen supply must match the physiologic demands. Too much oxygen can depress respiratory drive in a COPD patient. Dyspnea and RPE can be used to subjectively assess the amount of exertion and therefore the demand, where-as the pulse oximeter is a relatively economical and objective means of assessing oxygen demand. Initially, however, the oximeter should be correlated with the ABG values, because it is the $PaCO_2$ level, not oxygen saturation, that "plays tricks" on the respiratory center in the brainstem.

RECOMMENDED READINGS

ACSM: *Guidelines for exercise testing and prescription* (ed 6), Philadelphia: Lippincott Williams & Wilkins, 2000.

ACSM: *Resource manual for guidelines for exercise testing and prescription* (ed 4), Philadelphia: Lippincott Williams & Wilkins, 2001.

Carter R, Brooke N, Tucker JV: *Courage and information for life with chronic obstructive disease*, Onset, Mass: New Technology Publishing, 1999.

Hodgkin JE, Celli BR, Connors GL: *Pulmonary rehabilitation: guidelines to success*, Philadelphia: Lippincott Williams & Wilkins, 2000.

Weg JG, Hass CF: Long-term oxygen therapy for COPD: improving longevity and quality of life in hypoxemic patients, *Postgrad Med* 103:147, 1998.

American Physical Therapy Association: Guide to physical therapist practice, second edition, *Phys Ther* 81:1, 2001.

LEARNING OBJECTIVES

The reader will be able to:

1. Describe the elements of a musculoskeletal examination of the knee.
2. List and describe the signs, symptoms, and clinical patterns for the presence of a giant cell tumor.
3. Explain the importance of referring individuals to the appropriate specialist when there is any indication that the problem may be beyond the scope and expertise of the physical therapist.
4. Describe the appropriate interventions for an individual after bone and soft tissue surgery of the knee.

Examination

HISTORY

During a brisk 2-mile walk on her lunch break, a 27-year-old woman began to experience pain along the medial aspect of her left knee. She completed the walk and returned to work in her office for the remainder of the afternoon. Still feeling the pain in her left knee, she drove home from work in noticeable discomfort. Shortly after the woman got home, a neighbor dropped off the woman's 4-year-old daughter from daycare. The woman's husband, a self-employed building contractor, did not get home until 7 P.M. that evening. Meanwhile, she continued to ambulate and bear weight on the painful extremity while she prepared dinner for her family and cared for her daughter. She took two Tylenol for the pain, which was now a dull throbbing ache.

When her husband got home, the woman was finally able to get off her feet, sit down, and elevate her leg. The painful area was now visibly swollen. She decided to take a hot bath. The bath relaxed her and made her feel slightly better, but increased the swelling around her left knee and further restricted her active range of motion. She went to bed early, but the throbbing made it difficult to fall asleep, and she did not sleep well.

The next morning, the woman got up and decided to wrap her knee with an ace bandage. She took two more Tylenol and left for work. The pain didn't seem as bad as it did

the night before. She managed to get around the office by favoring her left leg and stopping to elevate her leg whenever possible. This pattern continued for several days before she finally decided to call her family physician.

The woman saw her doctor, who said she probably twisted her knee while walking. The doctor told her to stay off her feet as much as possible and gave her a prescription for Anaprox (a nonsteroidal antiinflammatory drug), which she took for the next 10 days. She felt better the next morning and continued her busy work and home schedule. A few days after her prescription ran out, the pain returned, and it progressively worsened over the next several days. She called her physician, who suggested that she see a physical therapist. The referral slip said, "mild sprain of the medial collateral ligament. Evaluate and treat."

SYSTEMS REVIEW

The physical therapist took a complete history, including the nature, onset, and location of the pain. The patient had no other pertinent medical history. An examination of cognitive, cardiovascular, pulmonary, neurologic, and integumentary systems was unremarkable.

The patient had an obvious limp as she walked and favored her left leg when she ambulated or stood still. This caused her to lean slightly to the right. Strength and joint range of motion were evaluated; the results are given in Table 32-1. The end feel for passive

**TABLE 32-1
STRENGTH/RANGE OF MOTION
DATA**

	(R) PROM	(R) MMT	(L) PROM	(L) MMT
Hip				
Flexion	0-120	5/5	0-120	4/5
Extension	0-30	5/5	0-30	4/5
Abduction	0-45	5/5	0-45	5/5
Adduction	0-30	5/5	0-30	5/5
Medial rotation	0-45	5/5	0-45	4/5
Lateral rotation	0-45	5/5	0-45	4/5
Knee				
Flexion	0-135	5/5	10-100	3/5
Extension	0-10	5/5	10	3/5
Ankle				
Dorsiflex	0-20	5/5	0-20	4/5
Plantarflex	0-50	5/5	0-50	5/5

L, Left; *R,* right; *MMT,* manual muscle test; *PROM,* passive range of motion.

range of motion (ROM) of the left knee was soft with pain in those movements demonstrating a limitation. Resistance during a manual muscle test (MMT) for flexion and extension of the involved knee also elicited a painful response. Tests for the integrity of the collateral and cruciate ligaments, and menisci were all negative.

The patient rated her pain on a visual analog scale as 5/10 in the morning and 8/10 at the end of a typical workday. Most nights it was intense enough (7/10) to disrupt her sleep.

Why did the physical therapist rule out the diagnosis of sprained medial collateral ligament?

Sensation, skin temperature, color, and peripheral pulses all appeared normal. The physical therapist noted that the patient had point tenderness over the medial tibial plateau and discovered a palpable soft mass on the medial aspect of the patient's left knee. The therapist explained the findings to the patient

and recommended that she be examined by an orthopedic surgeon. Her medical insurance plan required that she obtain a referral from her primary care physician. The therapist called the family physician and explained the findings, and an appointment was scheduled with the orthopedic surgeon.

To make the patient more comfortable, the physical therapist instructed her to continue to wrap the knee with an ace bandage, apply an ice pack, elevate her leg as much as possible, and use crutches. The therapist recommended that it would be prudent for the patient to ambulate non–weight-bearing until seen by the orthopedic specialist.

The orthopedic specialist's examination produced the same results that the physical therapist had observed, most notably, the presence of a soft palpable mass. The patient was sent for magnetic resonance imaging, which demonstrated the presence of a $3 \times 2 \times 2$ cm lesion in the left medial tibial plateau and extending outside the bone. The mass was causing the medial collateral ligament to bulge outward. A preliminary diagnosis of osteoclastomas, also known as giant cell tumor, was made at that time.

What allowed the orthopedic specialist to make the diagnosis of giant cell tumor so quickly?

Giant cell tumors are the most common bone tumor found in individuals between age 25 and 40. They are more common in females and usually found in the distal femur, proximal tibia and distal radius. Pain and swelling begin when the lesion begins to destroy the cortex of the bone and irritate the periosteum. About 85% of giant cell tumors are benign, but benign giant cell tumors can metastasize to the lungs. Treatment involves curettage of the tumor and bone graft replacement, or bone chip packing of the cavity left by removal of the tumor. A recurrence rate of 40% to 60% is seen in the first 2 years after surgery.

A lung scan and bone scan were performed to identify any other lesions; both were negative. The patient was discharged the day after surgery after being seen by the physical therapist in the hospital. She already had crutches and knew how to ambulate non–weight-bearing. Because of the bone loss from the lesion, a cast was applied, and the patient remained non–weight-bearing for 6 weeks. After 6 weeks, a radiograph was taken. The cast was removed and replaced with a lightweight brace for support. The patient was allowed to walk with crutches (partial weight bearing) for another month. When the cast was removed, the orthopedic surgeon referred the patient to the physical therapist once again.

Diagnosis

Physical Therapist Practice Pattern 4I: Impaired Joint Mobility, Motor Function, Muscle Performance, and Range of Motion Associated with Bony or Soft Tissue Surgery.

What was an appropriate physical therapy plan of care for this patient?

Prognosis

GOALS

The patient will:
1. Increase her aerobic capacity to 42 mL/kg/minute, which is above the 80th percentile for her age and gender, over a period of 4 to 6 weeks.
2. Increase her lower extremity muscle strength to 5/5 in the involved knee over a period of 4 to 6 weeks of exercise three times per week along with a daily home exercise program.
3. Increase her ROM for right knee flexion to 0 to 135 degrees and extension to 0 degrees during the same time frame required for muscle strengthening.

EXPECTED OUTCOME

The expected outcome will be attained during 4 to 6 weeks of outpatient physical therapy three times a week accompanied by a daily home exercise program. The patient's aerobic capacity will improve and muscle performance (strength, power and endurance) will increase. The patient will regain the ability to perform activities related to home management, work, and leisure.

DISCHARGE PLAN

The patient will be discharged from physical therapy when she had full passive and active ROM in the involved knee, muscle strength equal to the contralateral leg, and the ability to perform all activities of daily living at her previous level.

Intervention

After the physical therapist's reexamination, the patient was encouraged to perform gentle active range of motion exercises along with quadriceps and hamstring setting. When subsequent radiographs demonstrated complete bone healing, a more aggressive program for muscle strengthening and joint ROM was instituted.

She performed cardiovascular/pulmonary exercises on a bicycle ergometer, UBE, and walking at an appropriate intensity, beginning at 60% of the age-predicted maximum heart rate and progressing toward 90% as her fitness level increased. The program also included isometric, isokinetic, and isotonic exercises; heat application; and aquatic therapy.

Outcome

The patient increased her maximum aerobic capacity from 37 mL/kg/minute to 42 mL/kg/minute, as measured by bicycle ergometry. In addition, she increased strength in the involved extremity to 5/5. The giant cell tumor was removed with no recurrence. The pathology was corrected, and the patient had a full recovery with no residual impairments, disabilities, or handicaps.

Discussion

Giant cell tumors are common in women of this patient's age group. Most are discovered accidentally when patients are seen by a health care specialist for what appears to be a common musculoskeletal injury. If these patients are not seen, diagnosed, and treated promptly, the bone that has been weakened by the tumor will eventually fracture. As commonly seen, this patient had family and work responsibilities that caused her to delay seeking prompt treatment.

Because the physical therapist followed the *Guide to Physical Therapist Practice* and performed a thorough examination, the tumor was detected and the appropriate referral was made. Subsequently, the correct treatment was provided and the patient had a positive outcome. Had the physical therapist not detected the tumor, the patient likely would have received inappropriate care and delayed the appropriate intervention until she fractured her tibia and radiographs revealed the tumor. This case underscores the importance of a thorough and accurate examination.

RECOMMENDED READINGS

Dorfman HD, Czerniak B: *Bone tumors*, St Louis: Mosby, 1998.

Schubach GD, Wallis JW: Diagnosis: giant cell tumor, available at http://www.gamma.wvstl.edu/bs047tel143.html

ViaHealth: Bone disorders: giant cell tumor, available at http://www.viahealth.org/disease/bone-disorders/giant.html.

ACSM: *Guidelines for exercise testing and prescription* (ed 6), Philadelphia: Lippincott Williams & Wilkins, 2000.

American Physical Therapy Association: Guide to physical therapist practice, second edition, *Phys Ther* 81:1, 2001.

LEARNING OBJECTIVES

The reader will be able to:

1. Identify the preferred practice pattern for a patient who has undergone open reduction, internal fixation surgery on the hip.
2. Identify signs and symptoms indicating a lack of expected response to nitroglycerine medication.

Examination

A home health physical therapist was treating a 72-year-old man who was recovering from an open reduction internal fixation of a right hip fracture. The man had a history of angina and had non–insulin-dependent diabetes. He was ambulatory with the use of a walker and 50% weight bearing; he ambulated about his home without difficulty. The improvement in strength and ambulation the patient demonstrated indicated that he had been performing his exercises as directed.

Diagnosis

Physical Therapist Practice Pattern 4I: Impaired Joint Mobility, Motor Function, Muscle Performance, and Range of Motion Associated with Bony or Soft Tissue Surgery.

One morning, the therapist arrived to find the patient in bed and in moderate distress. The patient indicated that he woke at about 4 A.M. with tightness in the chest and periodic chest pains. He reported having slight difficulty with respiration. The patient's pulse rate was 96 beats per minute and blood pressure was 150/100 mm Hg, both measured with the patient supine. The patient indicated that he had taken his medication for diabetes and that his blood sugar level was within acceptable limits. Information gathered during the initial evaluation several weeks earlier indicated the patient also used nitroglycerin. The patient indicated he had taken nitroglycerin twice since 4 A.M., but that it had made no difference in his chest discomfort.

Evaluation

What was the immediate concern regarding the reported ineffectiveness of the medication?

Nitroglycerin is a fast-acting medication. Normally, a patient would notice some relief of chest discomfort almost immediately on taking the medication. The therapist examined the label on the medication bottle and found that the nitroglycerin prescription was 2 years beyond the indicated expiration date. Meanwhile, the patient became diaphoretic and exhibited increased difficulty breathing. He took another nitroglycerin tablet, but the medication failed to produce any change in symptoms.

What was the most appropriate course of action?

Intervention

This patient presented all the symptoms of an acute cardiac event. The therapist contacted emergency medical services, which then transferred the patient to the local hospital. During transport, the ambulance crew administered additional nitroglycerin. Within moments, the patient indicated that his chest pain had subsided substantially and he could breathe more easily.

Outcomes

After the patient's discharge from the hospital, it was determined that the nitroglycerin that he had been taking was old and ineffective. A therapist providing home health services needs to know the location of any medication that the patient is taking, so he or she can help provide that medication in the event of distress. In this case, the therapist's knowledge of the patient's home environment and the normally fast-acting nature of nitroglycerin was essential enabled the therapist to recognize a cardiac distress situation and initiate action. When the patient returned home, he was provided with a new supply of nitroglycerin tablets. He was also instructed by his physician to call for a new supply every 6 months.

Discussion

The therapist attempted to monitor the situation and contacted emergency medical services when all conservative measures had failed. The steps taken were appropriate for the situation. The important point in this case is the failure of the nitroglycerin to relieve symptoms. Nitroglycerin relaxes vascular smooth muscle, producing a general vasodilation effect throughout the body. The administration of nitroglycerin has been shown to reduce blood pressure in some patients. Pharmacists commonly suggest that nitroglycerin pills older than 6 months be discarded.

RECOMMENDED READINGS

Baumann BM, Perrone J, Hornig SE, et al: Randomized, double-blind, placebo-controlled trial of diazepam, nitroglycerin, or both for treatment of patients with potential cocaine-associated acute coronary syndromes, *Acad Emerg Med* 7:878, 2000.

Cooper A, Hodgkinson DW, Oliver RM: Chest pain in the emergency department, *Hosp Med* 61:178, 2000.

Engelberg S, Singer AJ, Moldashel J, et al: Effects of prehospital nitroglycerin on hemodynamics and chest pain intensity, *Prehosp Emerg Care* 4:290, 2000.

Everts B, Karlson B, Wahrbog P, et al: Pain recollection after chest pain of cardiac origin, *Cardiology* 92:115, 1999.

Kimble LP, Kunik CL: Knowledge and use of sublingual nitroglycerin and cardiac-related quality of life in patients with chronic stable angina, *J Pain Symptom Manage* 19:109, 2000.

Mahmarian JJ, Moye LA, Chinoy DA, et al: Transdermal nitroglycerin patch therapy improves left ventricular function and prevents remodeling after acute myocardial infarction: results of a multicenter prospective randomized, double-blind, placebo-controlled trial, *Circulation* 97:2017, 1999.

Purvis GM, Weiss SJ, Gaffney FA: Prehospital ECG monitoring of chest pain patients, *Am J Emerg Med* 17:604, 1999.

LEARNING OBJECTIVES

The reader will be able to:

1. Describe potential risks of personal contamination when performing wound debridement procedures.

2. Describe ways to reduce risks of personal contamination while performing wound debridement procedures.

Examination

HISTORY

Two physical therapists were assigned to work in the hydrotherapy department of an acute care hospital. For the past 2 weeks one of their interventions consisted of providing hydrotherapy to a very ill patient who was positive for human immunodeficiency virus (HIV) and hepatitis C and had open wounds. A large portion of the area receiving debridement was very painful and frequently bled into the whirlpool.

Diagnosis

Physical Therapist Practice Pattern 7D: Impaired Integumentary Integrity Associated with Full-Thickness Skin Involvement and Scar Formation.

The patient generally tolerated wound debridement well. In one particular instance, however, as a wound was being cleaned, the patient suddenly moved because of pain. The sudden movement, although completely accidental, splashed water into one therapist's face and directly into her eye. The therapist immediately dropped her debridement tools and jumped back, requesting a towel. The therapist did not suffer any puncture wounds from the sharp instruments she was holding at the time of the incident.

What was the best response in this situation?

Intervention

The first therapist calmed the patient and quickly came to the assistance of the therapist who had been splashed with the contaminated water. She helped wipe the therapist's face and then used an eye irrigation system available within the department to cleanse and irrigate the eye. Although no water had entered the therapist's mouth, the first therapist helped rinse the splashed therapist's mouth with 10% hydrogen peroxide. The splashed therapist was taken to the emergency department, where her eye was irrigated again and blood samples were taken to establish a baseline by which to monitor exposure to HIV.

Outcome

The accident was documented with an incident report. Since the splash incident, departmental policies and procedures have changed. The entire department was instructed in the proper mechanisms to use in the event of a similar incident. Anyone now working in the hydrotherapy department must wear a face shield to prevent another such event. To date, additional tests have been negative for the presence of HIV, and the therapist continues to work in the same hydrotherapy area. All health care workers exposed to any blood-borne pathogen should be baseline tested immediately after exposure.

Discussion

What health care concerns should therapists have when providing sharp instrument debridement?

Although there are no documented instances of a therapist contracting HIV through hydrotherapy, exposure safety precautions must be followed. Besides wearing proper clothing, it is important to add chemical disinfectants to the water to lessen the probability of exposure should a splash occur. In this instance, the water had been treated with chemical disinfectants before the initiation of debridement.

HIV is not the only transmissible virus of concern to healthcare providers. Hepatitis C, a viral disease primarily affecting the liver, has infected more than 4 million people in the United States. Worldwide, it affects an estimated 3% of the population. It has been projected that up to 10,000 people in the United States will die each year from the disease, and that this death toll may triple by the year 2010. The primary transmission route for hepatitis C is through the blood. The risk to health care workers for contracting hepatitis C by needle stick is between 1.2% and 10%, compared with 0.3% for HIV. Appropriate safety procedures must always be taken by therapists during hydrotherapy to avoid puncture wounds with sharp and potentially contaminated instruments.

RECOMMENDED READINGS

Beekmann SE, Vaughn TE, McCoy KD, et al: Hospital bloodborne pathogens programs: program characteristics and blood and body fluid exposure rates, *Infect Control Hosp Epidemiol* 22:73, 2001.

Berrouane YF, McNutt LA, Buschelman BJ, et al: Outbreak of severe *Pseudomonas aeruginosa* infections caused by a contaminated drain in a whirlpool bathtub, *Clin Infect Dis* 31:1331, 2000.

Burke DT, Ho CH, Saucier MA, Stewart G: Effects of hydrotherapy on pressure ulcer healing, *Am J Phys Med Rehabil* 77:394, 1998.

Dillman CM: Hepatitis C: a danger to healthcare workers, *Nurs Forum* 34:23, 1999.

Ganju SA, Goel A: Prevalence of HBV and HCV infection among health care workers (HCWs), *J Commum Dis* 32:228, 2000.

Gogi PP: Physical therapy modalities for wound management, *Ostomy Wound Manage* 42:46, 50, 54, 1996.

Hollyoak V, Boyd P, Freeman R: Whirlpool baths in nursing homes: use, maintenance, and contamination with *Pseudomonas aeruginosa*, *Commun Dis Rep CDR Rev* 23:102, 1995.

Juve Meeker B: Whirlpool therapy on postoperative pain and surgical wound healing: an exploration, *Patient Educ Couns* 33:39, 1998.

Madan AK, Rentz DE, Wahle MJ, Flint LM: Noncompliance of health care workers with universal precautions during trauma resuscitations, *South Med J* 94:277, 2001.

Moloughney BW: Transmission and postexposure management of bloodborne virus infections in the health care setting: where are we now? *CMAJ* 165:445, 2001.

Pearson T: The wearing of facial protection in high-risk environments, *Br J Perioper Nurs* 10:163, 2000.

Stevens AB, Coyle PV: Hepatitis C virus: an important occupational hazard? *Occup Med (Lond)* 50:377, 2000.

LEARNING OBJECTIVES

The reader will be able to:

1. Define the "terrible triad" injury.
2. Discuss a possible cause for a joint infection.
3. Describe signs and symptoms of a joint infection.

The reader should know that a 23-year-old man had been referred to physical therapy after sustaining an injury to his right knee while playing intramural basketball 1 week earlier. The patient was initially treated in a hospital emergency department and referred to an orthopedic surgeon for specialist care. The patient was seen the next day by an orthopedic surgeon, who aspirated about 20 mL of blood from the knee. The injury was sustained when the patient was rebounding and felt the knee give way when he came down with the ball. The physician suspected the "terrible triad" injury, to the medial collateral ligament, medial meniscus, and the anterior cruciate ligament. The patient desired to attempt physical therapy for a period of time before agreeing to arthroscopic surgery or any form of reconstruction. On examination, the therapist found the patient bearing partial weight on the leg while using crutches. The knee was very warm and sensitive to light touch, and range of motion was painful, with flexion to only 70 degrees and extension limited to –15 degrees. The patient indicated he had been running a low-grade fever of 99 degrees and that he generally was not feeling well. The physician requested a physical therapist initiate range of motion (ROM) and progress weight-bearing as tolerated. The first intervention (consisting of gentle ROM) did not go well, because the patient was experiencing severe pain. The patient made no discernible progress in obtaining additional ROM.

Examination

HISTORY

The patient was a physically well-conditioned young man who had been running and working out in a gym regularly. He indicated that he weighed 225 pounds and was capable of bench-pressing 300 pounds and squat-lifting 400 pounds. He reported that he played college football and had sustained injuries in the past but none to this degree. None of the previous injuries involved the lower extremities. Medications included a nonsteroidal antiinflammatory drug and a mild pain reliever. He took pain medication before attending the first physical therapy session. He believed he had good pain tolerance. He stated that he had been accepted to law school and was planning to begin school in 8 months.

SYSTEMS REVIEW

The patient presented with no known cardiac or pulmonary problems. His heart rate was within normal limits. Blood pressure was 150/90 mm Hg, measured in the left upper extremity while seated. The patient indicated that his blood pressure was usually much lower, and he believed that it was high because the pain in his leg had kept him awake the night before.

TESTS AND MEASURES

Sensation was intact throughout the lower extremity. ROM and strength were within normal limits in the involved hip and ankle. The knee was visibly swollen and warm to the touch. Palpation to the soft tissues around the knee elicited a very painful response. The patient indicated he had been applying ice once an hour for 20 minutes, but that the knee "just heats right back up." There was no reported calf discomfort or pain on palpation.

What type of problem was suspected?

Evaluation

The therapist recognized the problem as possibly related to an infection in the knee joint. The knee was warm and sensitive to light touch. The patient indicated he had a good pain tolerance and had been applying ice to the area as recommended. The calf presented no tenderness upon palpation.

Diagnosis

Physical Therapist Practice Pattern 4E: Impaired Joint Mobility, Motor Function, Muscle Performance, and Range of Motion Associated with Localized Inflammation.

What was an appropriate course of action?

Intervention

The physician's office was immediately contacted and apprised of the patient's symptoms. The patient was seen by the physician later that same day and subsequently admitted to the hospital. The next day the patient underwent arthroscopic surgery for knee irrigation and was given intravenous antibiotics for 7 days. It was suspected the patient may have contracted a staphylococcal infection of the knee during needle aspiration of the joint.

Outcome

Once the infection was under control, the patient resumed physical therapy. The primary goal of rehabilitation was to restore ROM and ambulation. Because of the presence of the infection, no attempt was made by the surgeon to make internal derangement repairs to the knee. Repairs were performed at a later date once there was convincing evidence that the infection had subsided. The patient resumed ambulation without gait abnormalities and began law school. His conditioning program now included a low-weight, high-repetition program for the involved extremity.

RECOMMENDED READINGS

Dubost JJ, Soubrier M, Sauvezie B: Pyogenic arthritis in adults, *Joint Bone Spine* 67:11, 2000.

Holder-Powell HM, DiMatteo G, Rutherford OM: Do knee injuries have long-term consequences for isometric and dynamic muscle strength? *Eur J Appl Physiol* 85:310, 2001.

Hurley MV: The effects of joint damage on muscle function, proprioception and rehabilitation, *Man Ther* 2:11, 1997.

Le Dantec L, Maury F, Flipo RM, et al: Peripheral pyogenic arthritis: a study of one hundred seventy-nine cases. *Rev Rhum Engl Ed* 63:103, 1996.

Nair SP, Williams RJ, Henderson B: Advances in our understanding of the bone and joint pathology caused by *Staphylococcus aureus* infection, *Rheumatology (Oxford)* 39:821, 2000.

Regev A, Weinberger M, Fishman M, et al: Necrotizing fasciitis caused by *Staphylococcus aureus*, *Eur J Clin Microbiol Infect Dis* 17:101, 1998.

Smerdelj M, Pecina M, Hasp M: Surgical treatment of infected knee contracture after war injury, *Acta Med Croatica* 54:151, 2000.

Solomom DH, Simel DL, Bates DW, et al: Does this patient have a torn meniscus or ligament of the knee? Value of the physical examination, *JAMA* 286:1610, 2001.

Swain R: An unusual cause of knee pain in an adolescent basketball player, *Clin J Sport Med* 10:142, 2000.

Case 36

LEARNING OBJECTIVES

The reader will be able to:

1. Discuss the importance of history taking as an ongoing process.

2. Describe appropriate procedures to follow when spontaneous bleeding occurs during physical therapy (whirlpool) intervention.

Examination

A therapist was assigned to hydrotherapy to fill in for another therapist who had to attend an unscheduled mandatory meeting in another area of the hospital. That therapist indicated that the patient had a full-thickness third-degree burn involving the anterior compartment of the left lower extremity. The extremity also had an infection with *Staphyloccocus aureus* that was seriously affecting the healing of a recent surgical skin graft. To fully irrigate the wound, the patient had to lie semireclined in a full-body whirlpool. Sterile technique was to be followed throughout the course of the treatment. The patient's entire medical record and rehabilitative service records were available for review before initiating intervention. The patient received hydrotherapy twice daily.

The patient sustained the burn as a result of falling asleep in bed while smoking. He had been to surgery on two occasions. The first surgery was after admission to the hospital for wound debridement. The second surgical intervention occurred 12 days after the first operation once the wound was ready for grafting. During that surgery 5 days earlier, grafts were taken from donor sites on both thighs.

The patient was receiving intravenous (IV) antibiotics, intramuscular (IM) morphine for pain relief, and coumadin (an anticoagulant) because of concerns regarding potential phlebitis. The IV site, located in the right forearm, had required replacement twice because the patient exposed the arm to the whirlpool water, loosening the tape and partially removing the needle. The patient's most pressing health care concern was, however, the potential loss of the grafts as a result of infection.

The patient was a 61-year-old man who was a heavy smoker (41 years of two packs per day) and had little formal education. He lived alone and indicated he had no interest in stopping smoking. He was cooperative but seldom understood complex medical terms and concepts. A review of the chart indicated that he had signed all consent forms by marking an "X" in areas for signature.

The patient's physician requested aggressive cleansing of the wound. Small superficial pockets of purulent drainage were present, and the patient had a low-grade fever of 101° F. Additionally, to enhance wound healing, the physician requested that staples with overgrowing skin be removed.

Evaluation

The patient was a suitable candidate for physical therapy intervention. He received whirlpool twice daily and was receiving the first of two scheduled sessions. Thirty minutes before the whirlpool treatment, he received intramuscularly administered pain medication. Without this medication, the patient could not tolerate treatment intervention and became impatient and agitated. Timing whirlpool sessions in conjunction with the administration of pain medication was critical to providing effective whirlpool interventions.

Diagnosis

Physical Therapist Practice Pattern 7D: Impaired Integumentary Integrity Associated with Full-Thickness Skin Involvement and Scar Formation.

Intervention

While cleaning the wound, the therapist came across a staple near the surface of the skin that was particularly difficult to remove. When removed, blood suddenly began pulsating from the leg while the extremity was under water.

What was the proper response to the bleeding?

The patient in this case had been receiving physical therapy since his hospital admission. Before initiating an intervention with this patient, the therapist had thoroughly reviewed the patient's chart. Part of this review included reading earlier therapy notes, nursing notes, and notes on the surgeries that had been performed. The therapist also spoke in depth with the patient regarding his response to intervention and how he believed he was progressing. Because of the patient's inability to ambulate, his physician had become concerned regarding the potential for phlebitis in the lower extremities and had initiated coumadin therapy 4 days earlier. The therapist informed the patient of the importance of anticoagulant medication and its potential impact on intervention. Rehabilitative services support staff directly involved in providing care to the patient were apprised of the potential change in the patient's health care status and the new medication. Because of the patient's fever, the therapist informed support staff that the typical duration of whirlpool therapy may have to be decreased if the patient indicates that he is not feeling well.

Staple removal must always be done with caution. It is not uncommon for small arterioles to bleed as a result of stress caused by wound care in adjacent areas. Clotting ability may be reduced with the addition of coumadin. Arterial bleeding near the surface of the skin is often best controlled with direct pressure. In this case, the correct response was to leave the patient in the whirlpool. The combination of pressure of the water in the whirlpool and direct pressure applied with a gauze bandage controlled the bleeding. Keeping the patient in the whirlpool and applying pressure to the wound allowed others to make arrangements to transfer the patient to a stretcher for rapid transport, if needed. In this case the wound stopped bleeding, and the session was safely concluded.

Based on the occurrence of bleeding in the first whirlpool session, was it appropriate to cancel the second scheduled session?

The therapist decided to proceed with the afternoon session of whirlpool intervention, but did not proceed as aggressively with debridement. The session went well, and the patient tolerated the intervention with minimal bleeding.

Outcomes

The preferred method to control severe bleeding is the application of direct pressure. In the absence of a compress, a gloved hand or fingers may be used, but only until a compress pad can be applied. Blood clots should not be disturbed once they have formed. If blood soaks through the entire pad without clotting, then the pad should not be removed; instead, additional thick layers of dressing should be added and direct pressure continued. If pressure firmly applied to the area does not assist in the control of bleeding, then the extremity should be elevated and pressure also applied to the artery supplying the involved area. In this case, direct pressure was applied to the site with gauze while the extremity remained in the whirlpool. The wound stopped bleeding within 2 minutes of pressure application without harm to the patient.

Discussion

Beyond the issues regarding successful wound care management, this case presents issues concerning the proper steps to take when following previous health care interventions and providers. A patient with a third-degree burn grafting and infection may demonstrate changes in health care status between therapy interventions. In this case the therapist not only reviewed the patient's chart but also spent significant time gaining an understanding of how the diagnosis and previous interventions may have changed since the last whirlpool session. Because of the therapist's interest in understanding the current health status of the patient, there was no surprise when the prescribed medication increased the likelihood of bleeding. Providing whirlpool intervention as a follow-up to other health care interventions requires the therapist to collect and sort new data that can identify potential problems and improve outcome potential.

What was a reasonable health care "team approach" concerning patient education?

Fires started by cigarettes are the most common source of fatal house fires. Approximately 29% of fire deaths in the United States are caused in a manner similar to how this patient was burned. With limited ambulation ability and a refusal to stop smoking, this patient was at risk for further injury. The focus of the patient education effort became one of involving social services, the physician, and the physical therapist in an educational effort to assist the patient in lifestyle modification. The physical therapy program included improving the patient's overall conditioning. Social services focused on encouraging the patient to attend a local smoking cessation program. The physician emphasized to the patient the need to stop smoking to maintain good oxygenation levels in order to promote proper wound healing. Over the next several months, the patient was able to reduce his smoking significantly and achieved good wound healing.

RECOMMENDED READINGS

Barillo DJ, Brigham PA, Kayden DA, et al: The fire-safe cigarette: a burn-prevention tool, *J Burn Care Rehabil* 21:162, 2000.

Fritsch DE, Coffee TL, Yowler CJ: Characteristics of burn patients developing pressure ulcers, *J Burn Care Rehabil* 22:293, 2001.

Ho WS, Ying SY, Chan HH: A study of burn injuries in the elderly in a regional burn center, *Burns* 27:382, 2001.

Muller MJ, Pegg SP, Rile MR: Determinants of death following burn injury, *Br J Surg* 88:583, 2001.

Stassen NA, Lukan JK, Mizuguchi NN, et al: Thermal injury in the elderly: when is comfort care the right choice? *Am Surg* 67:704, 2001.

Stiles NJ, Bratcher D, Ramsbottom-Lucier M, Hunter G: Evaluating fire safety in older persons through home visits, *J Ky Med Assoc* 99:105, 2001.

Treharne LJ, Kay AR: The initial management of acute burns, *J R Army Med Corps* 147:198, 2001.

Wibbenmeyer LA, Amelon MJ, Morgan LJ, et al: Predicting survival in an elderly patient population, *Burns* 27:583, 2001.

LEARNING OBJECTIVES

The reader will be able to:

1. Identify and recommend creative switch placement for use of assistive technology for children/consumers whose physical disabilities limit the use of more conventional switch solutions.

2. Differentiate between criteria/candidacy for contemporary spasticity management alternatives.

Examination

HISTORY

The patient was an 11-year-old white male with choreoathetotic and spastic cerebral palsy, who was significantly compromised in movement and physical interactions with his environment. Electronic devices (i.e., for communication and mobility) had the potential to improve his participation in home and school environments. Evolution of assistive technology switch choices, including type and placement, to facilitate interaction with his environment, had been slow and frustrating for the child, his parents, and his younger sibling.

This child first demonstrated atypical motor skill development at age 4 months. He exhibited significant limitations in movement, mobility, and access to his environment because of his athetoid movements, spasticity, and muscle spasms. The child found it difficult to maintain a seated position because of hypertonicity, and he began to arch and slide, requiring frequent assistance with repositioning. Furthermore, spasms were a problem during the day and night, and his sleep was frequently disrupted because of apparent discomfort.

SYSTEMS REVIEW

Initial observation showed a thin child in no apparent distress. Musculoskeletal examination revealed limited flexibility in the hamstrings bilaterally. This child reported lower extremity pain, specifically in the left hip on passive or active movement, and his position of comfort was with the left hip in flexion, adduction, and internal rotation, accompanied by knee flexion. Other findings included hypertonicity in the extremities and athetoid movements in the upper extremities and oral-motor musculature. Neuromuscular examination revealed that the child had a floor mobility strategy using side-to-side rolling. He maintained short sitting when placed and provided with maximal adult assistance at the trunk. He required adult assistance for all transfer and positioning tasks.

The child's cognitive skill level was close to age level, and he attended school in the community in which he lived. He had experienced significant limitations in movement, access, and mobility because of his athetoid movements, spasticity, and muscle spasms. He made several verbal utterances ("yeah," for example), but otherwise communicated using a DynaMyte augmentative communication device (Dynavox Systems, Sunrise Medical, Pittsburgh, Pennsylvania), using an automatic scan setting. With that setting, the device scrolled through categories of topics, from which the user actively selected. Within the categories, the device had preprogrammed sentences, phrases, words, or responses. The individual waited for the device to advance to the desired response. (This child required switch access for both his augmentative communication device and his power wheelchair.) Since the child's preschool years, a long progression of switches had been implemented and abandoned, including a simple pad switch (or "jellybean") and toggle switches. Placement had also varied over the years, including upper extremity, lower extremity, head, and chin. All had been unsuccessful for long-term use.

TESTS AND MEASURES

Hamstring flexibility was measured with the hip positioned in 90 degrees of flexion and neutral rotation. The right knee lacked 30 degrees of extension, and the left knee lacked 45 degrees. Limitations of range of motion were noted, specifically hip extension on the left at –35 degrees (with discomfort), hip abduction on the right at 0 to 15 degrees, and hip abduction on the left at 0 to 5 degrees.

Muscle tone was evaluated using a modified Ashworth scale,[1] which provides specific criteria with which to evaluate spasticity. Muscle tone was graded on an ordinal scale of 0, 1, 1+, 2, 3, and 4, with 0 indicating no increase in muscle tone on imposition of quick stretch, 1 indicating a slight increase in muscle tone with a quick catch and release palpated (with *catch* defined as the initial resistance to motion in the muscle and *release* defined as subsequent muscle relaxation that permits motion), 1+ indicating a slight increase in muscle tone with a quick catch and release palpated and minimal resistance palpated through the remainder of the range of motion after the catch, 2 indicating more marked increase in muscle tone through much of the range of motion but with the affected part easily moved, 3 indicating considerable increase in muscle tone with passive movement difficult, and 4 indicating rigidity of flexion or extension in the affected part. Upper extremity tone was scored as 2 in the biceps and 3-4 in the triceps brachii; lower extremity muscle tone, as 3-4 in the adductors and hamstring muscles and 2 in the gastrosoleus complex. Variable muscle tone was reported, representing the range of findings in the described muscles during the physical examination.

The child's functional skill level was assessed using the Gross Motor Functional Classification System (GMFCS).[2] This ordinal classification scale measures a child's performance based on self-initiated movement. It is a five-level system, with distinctions between levels based on functional limitations and the individual's use of assistive technology, including a broad range of assistive and mobility devices. Level I describes motor function of those most mildly involved children, and level V represents motor function of children with severe limitations in self-mobility. This system is appropriate in evaluating individuals up to age 12. The patient in this case met the criteria for level V. Given the problems with selection of switch type and placement, the child's self-mobility was severely limited even with the use of assistive technology.

Evaluation

This child needed a switch that would use his most available motor strategy to activate the mobility and communication devices. The optimal placement for a switch would allow him to use movements over which he has the greatest control.

What considerations were incorporated into decisions regarding switch access for this individual?

A second major issue for this child centered on optimal management of spasticity. His spasticity influenced ease of positioning, ease of care, function, and comfort, which of course hindered his ability to participate maximally in his home, school, and community environments. Therapy with diazepam (Valium) had been used with some minimal appreciable effect. Because of the generalized distribution of his spasticity, the patient did not appear to be an appropriate candidate for botulinum toxin type A injections. Botulinum toxin type A has been described in the literature as producing the best effects when spasticity is focal versus generalized.[3] The patient also did not meet the criteria for selective dorsal rhizotomy.[4]

What were appropriate spasticity management options for discussion and potential trial?

Diagnosis

Physical Therapist Practice Pattern 5C: Impaired Motor Function and Sensory Integrity Associated with Nonprogressive Disorders of the Central Nervous System—Congenital Origin or Acquired in Infancy or Childhood.

Prognosis

Given appropriate switch placement and effective interface with mobility and communication systems, this child's prognosis predicted independent mobility in his school, home, and community environments (although he would continue to require adult assistance for transfers). Additionally, he was expected to attain an improved level of autonomy in communication because of the use of the switch (although this is outside of a physical therapist's scope of practice).

Intrathecal baclofen therapy was recommended by the spasticity management evaluation team. In this approach to reducing spasticity, the drug baclofen is introduced into the subarachnoid space through a catheter, which is attached to a computer-controlled pump.[5,6] This pump contains a reservoir for the drug and is refilled periodically. After a successful trial (using a bolus dose of baclofen, injected intrathecally), an intrathecal baclofen pump was implanted subcutaneously in the anterior abdominal wall. The child was expected to experience reduced spasticity and improved ease of positioning, with the benefits of a reduced burden of care for his caregivers and an improved ability to work toward independent sitting. Reduced pain and positional discomfort were also predicted.

After baclofen administration, what components of the physical therapy plan of care were considered?

The recommended plan of care included flexibility exercises, balance and posture awareness training, neuromotor development, strength training, intrathecal baclofen trial, and alternative switch trials. This child's school-based physical therapy program was provided three times per week, and status and outcomes were reevaluated at the end of the school year.

GOALS

Short-term goals included:
1. Improve hip abduction range of motion by 10 degrees to improve seated base of support, in 3 months.
2. Improve abdominal and erector spinae strength, for improved upright posture in sitting, measured at grade 3+, in 3 months.
3. Demonstrate success with powered mobility using appropriate switch, 80% of trials, in 6 months.
4. Demonstrate success with DynaMyte using appropriate switch, 80% of trials, in 6 months.
5. Demonstrate success with independent transfers between devices using appropriate switch, 80% of trials, evaluated in 6 months.

Long-term goals were as follows:
1. Maintain independent sitting, when on a firm surface, with close supervision, up to 5 minutes, in 6 months.
2. Demonstrate independent powered mobility in 100% of trials, in all environments, in 1 year.
3. Demonstrate independent communication using DynaMyte 100% of trials, in all environments, in 1 year.

How was evidence applied to guide selection of appropriate interventions?

Intervention

After numerous trials with prototypes using the creative input and suggestions of many team members and vendors, one long-term, useful solution for this child involved an infrared switch. This switch was mounted to a head set, an arrangement that finally provided the child with significantly greater consistency of switch access to his power wheelchair and DynaMyte augmentative communication device. The child used an oral-motor point of access (his area of greatest motor control) by interrupting the infrared beam with his tongue. He used this switch with considerable success, and continued to work on his accuracy and control using the switch with his wheelchair. Through problem-solving efforts of his assistive technology service providers, this one-of-a-kind prototype was created.

After a trial of oral baclofen and a trial bolus dose of baclofen intrathecally (both were successful), this child underwent an intrathecal baclofen pump insertion. He received this several months after his eleventh birthday.

Left hip radiograph findings indicated valgus positioning of the femoral neck-shaft relationship, with mild uncovering, but revealed nothing acute. The left femoral head was less developed than the right, but no significant signs of any displacement were noted. Non-steroidal antiinflammatory drugs were recommended[6] to reduce the child's discomfort related to any soft tissue or joint surface microtrauma and/or inflammation.

Reexamination

The child recently experienced switch failure, noted when the switch stopped functioning, because of suspected problems with excessive moisture (i.e., saliva). The switch was replaced. As a result of the switch failure, investigation into alternative switches using similar access is under way.

During evaluation after the baclofen pump implantation surgery, the child was noted to sit apparently quite comfortably in his wheelchair, with his right leg casually flexed, abducted, and crossed over the left. Evaluation of spasticity in the lower extremities (i.e., hip and knee musculature) using the modified Ashworth scale showed a reduction in scores ranging from 3 to 4 before pump implantation to 2 to 3 after pump implantation. When positioned in sitting on the edge of the examination table, the child maintained an upright position for several minutes with moderate trunk support. He showed no arching or sliding while maintaining this position.

Outcome

The patient's family reports that the patient is doing well, exhibiting a general reduction in muscle tone and pain. The family notes this subjectively, from their observations while assisting the child with activities of daily living. Reduced spasticity has also been noted on clinical examination. Functionally, the child shows improved participation in sitting, requiring less assistance and with greater relative comfort.

The child continues to work on consistency with independent mobility and maneuverability over greater distances, in the school setting, at this time. Efforts continue to fabricate a switch for the child that will have greater durability over time.

Although the child continues to complain about the left hip pain, before the pump he was frequently reported to hurt "everywhere." As the child experiences less discomfort, he will have greater attention and energy for tasks and challenges facing him daily.

REFERENCES

1. Bohannon RW, Smith MB: Interrater reliability of a modified Ashworth scale of muscle spasticity, *Phys Ther* 67:206, 1987.
2. Palisano R, Rosenbaum P, Walter S, et al: Development and reliability of a system to classify gross motor function of children with cerebral palsy, *Dev Med Child Neurol* 39:214, 1997.
3. Russman BS, Tilton A, Gormley ME: Cerebral palsy: a rational approach to a treatment protocol, and the role of botulinum toxin in treatment, *Muscle Nerve Suppl* 6:S181, 1997.
4. McLaughlin JF, Bjornson KF, Astley SJ, et al: Selective dorsal rhizotomy: efficacy and safety in an investigator-masked randomized clinical trial, *Dev Med Child Neurol* 40:220, 1998.
5. Campbell SK, Almeida GL, Penn RD, Corcos DM: The effects of intrathecally administered baclofen on function in patients with spasticity, *Phys Ther* 75:352, 1995.
6. Ciccone CD: *Pharmacology in rehabilitation* (ed 3), Philadelphia: FA Davis, 2001.

LEARNING OBJECTIVES

The reader will be able to:

1. Identify a reason why a patient may have anterior thigh pain after total hip arthroplasty surgery.
2. Discuss examination procedures to help identify the source of pain in a patient who has undergone total hip arthroplasty.
3. Formulate a recommendation for a patient status post–total hip arthroplasty with a residual leg length difference.

Examination

HISTORY

The patient, a 67-year-old man, requested a physical therapy examination of his right hip 6 months after undergoing total hip arthroplasty surgery. The patient indicated that he continued to experience leg pain, primarily in the anterior mid-thigh. According to the patient, he received extensive postsurgical physical therapy at a rehabilitation center for 1 month. That center provided him with an excellent home program, which he continued to perform with little or no difficulty. With his physician's approval, the patient progressed to working out three times a week at a local fitness center.

During the physical therapy examination, the patient ambulated with no assistive devices but exhibited a slight limp involving the right lower extremity. The patient reported that pain increased with prolonged ambulation and that the limp worsened the more he ambulated. He exhibited good passive and active hip range of motion. Strength in the right lower extremity was not equal to that in the left lower extremity, but there was no evidence of a Trendelenburg deviation that would contribute to the limp. The patient had only minimal soreness on palpation of the involved right hip and thigh. There were no reports of low back pain, and the knee and ankle presented full pain-free range of motion. At the conclusion of the examination the patient became frustrated and asked, "I'm returning to my doctor next week. Is there anything I should point out that might be helpful in addressing this problem?"

The patient was active in a number of outdoor recreational pursuits, and enjoyed camping, hiking, and swimming. Five years ago he had a lumbar fusion at L5-S1. He completed 6 weeks of physical therapy after the lumbar surgery. He indicated that he had one alcoholic beverage per day, usually with dinner. He reported no other significant surgeries, and his last physical examination, before the surgery, gave him a "clean bill of health."

SYSTEMS REVIEW

The patient presented with no cardiac or respiratory problems. His blood pressure was medication-controlled and within normal limits. Sensation was intact throughout.

TESTS AND MEASURES

Recently completed postoperative blood work ordered by the physician demonstrated all values within normal limits. Radiograph reports indicated good postoperative positioning of the prosthesis. The patient denied any history of hip dislocations.

What was another area of examination considered by the therapist?

Pain continued in the involved extremity and there was no possibility of a fracture; thus the therapist examined the patient for possible differences in leg length. In this case, the patient presented a difference of approximately

½ inch (12.7 mm), with the right leg shorter than the left. When questioned, the patient replied he had no idea that such a difference in length existed. The therapist who had provided the initial intervention apparently had not informed the patient of the leg length difference.

Diagnosis

Physical Therapist Practice Pattern 4H: Impaired Joint Mobility, Motor Function, Muscle Performance, and Range of Motion Associated With Joint Arthroplasty.

Intervention

If a true leg length difference is present, the therapist can recommend that the patient use a shoe lift or insert to correct the problem. Once the device fits properly, additional therapy is seldom required.

What was the therapist's recommendation to the patient's surgeon?

Outcome

Despite the efforts of every orthopedic surgeon to ensure leg length equality, obtaining equal leg lengths can be difficult. Surgeons often inform their patients that every effort will be made to ensure equal length, but that steps can be taken after the operation if a difference is present. Many surgeons assess for the presence of a difference in leg length only after several weeks of ambulation. The reason that surgeons prefer to wait is that a small difference in leg length may pose no problems to the patient.

In this case the therapist sent a note to the physician asking that consideration be given to providing an insert to see if the problem with pain during ambulation could be eliminated. The surgeon agreed with the recom-

mendation, and the patient was provided with an insert. Within 2 weeks, the patient was ambulating pain free. The patient subsequently had all of his shoes adjusted with permanent ½-inch lifts, and reported no further difficulties.

RECOMMENDED READINGS

Chaudhuri S, Aruin AS: The effect of shoe lifts on static and dynamic postural control in individuals with hemiparesis, *Arch Phys Med Rehabil* 81:1498, 2000.

Chiu HC, Chern JY, Chen SH, Chang JK: Physical functioning and health-related quality of life: before and after total hip replacement, *Kaohsiung J Med Sci* 16:285, 2000.

Chiu HC, Mau LW, Hsu YC, Chang JK: Postoperative 6-month and 1-year evaluation of health-related quality of life in total hip replacement patients, *J Formos Med Assoc* 100:461, 2001.

Garellick G, Malchau H, Herberts P, et al: Life expectancy and cost utility after total hip replacement, *Clin Orthop* 346:141, 1998.

Jones CA, Voaklander DC, Johnston DW, Suarez-Almazor ME: The effect of age on pain, function, and quality of life after total hip and knee arthroplasty, *Arch Intern Med* 161:454, 2001.

Knutsson S, Engberg IB: An evaluation of patients' quality of life before, 6 weeks and 6 months after total hip replacement, *J Adv Nurs* 30:1349, 1999.

March LM, Cross MJ, Lapsley H, et al: Outcomes after hip or knee replacement surgery for osteoarthritis: a prospective cohort study comparing patients' quality of life before and after surgery with age-related population norms, *Med J Aust* 171:235, 1999.

Ranawat CS, Rao RR, Rodriguez JA, Bhende HS: Correction of limb-length during total hip arthroplasty, *J Arthroplasty* 16:715, 2001.

Shields RK, Enloe LJ, Leo KC: Health-related quality of life in patients with total hip or knee replacement, *Arch Phys Med Rehabil* 80:572, 1999.

Towheed TE, Hochberg MC: Health-related quality of life after total hip replacement, *Semin Arthritis Rheum* 26:483, 1996.

LEARNING OBJECTIVES

The reader will be able to:

1. Describe the relationship between cast immobilization and possible peripheral nerve compression.

2. Discuss reasons why a patient may refuse gait training.

The reader should know that a therapist was asked to instruct a patient at bedside in crutch ambulation before the patient was discharged from the hospital. The patient was a 17-year-old male who sustained a right nondisplaced tibial plateau fracture the night before while playing a high school football game. The patient was struck slightly below the knee between the fibula and tibia. Most of the force was inflicted by a football helmet striking the tibia and the soft tissue area between the tibia and fibula. Radiographs were negative for a fibula fracture. The tibia fracture did not appear to have disrupted the growth plate. There was, however, a very strong possibility that he sustained internal derangement of the right knee. The patient was known as a top college running back prospect and was informed by his physician that he would not be able to play for the rest of the season.

Throughout the night, the patient made continual requests for pain medication. He was also very difficult for the orthopedic nursing staff to manage. The patient was angry over his situation and did not want to be bothered. His orthopedic physician had not seen him since applying a full leg cast in the emergency department at 11 P.M.

The patient was in significant pain and subsequently had refused to ambulate. Overnight, the leg had been elevated and externally rotated on two pillows with an ice pack applied to the site of the fracture. The foot was swollen, and the patient reported numbness over the dorsum of the foot. The patient was requested by the therapist to flex and extend his toes. The patient responded by flexing the toes, but toe extension could not be seen or palpated. The patient abruptly responded, "I've had enough, I'm not getting up, it hurts too much. Please just leave me alone!"

Examination

HISTORY

The patient was from a very poor socioeconomic background. According to the attending orthopedic nurse, the patient's family and home situation was known to be very difficult. The parents were not present during the initial physical therapy examination but were expected to arrive at the hospital 2 to 3 hours later to take their son home.

SYSTEMS REVIEW

The patient presented with no cardiac or pulmonary problems. His heart rate, blood pressure, and respiratory rate were within normal limits. Range of motion of the uninvolved lower extremity was within normal limits. The involved knee was casted to approximately 40 degrees flexion. Strength in the upper and the noninvolved lower extremities was within normal limits. Sensation in the areas above the cast, where palpation could be performed, was within normal limits. Sensation on the plantar surface of the toes was intact.

TESTS AND MEASURES

Active toe flexion was within normal limits. There was no evidence of active toe extension despite repeated attempts to elicit voluntary movement. Toe position sense was present, but sensation was markedly decreased on the dorsum of all toes.

Evaluation

Was it appropriate to consider the presence of an anterior compartment syndrome?

A compartment syndrome occurs when the circulation and function of muscle within a closed fascia space are compromised by increased pressure within that space. Blunt trauma can produce an acute compartment syndrome. Rapid clinical diagnosis and treatment is crucial to the prevention of complications associated with the condition.

Proximal-third tibia fractures account for 5% to 11% of all tibial shaft injuries. Treatment is typically more challenging, and the rate of compartment syndrome is higher, in distal tibia fractures. If an acute compartment syndrome is present, then fasciotomy is generally required to relieve the pressure and restore neurologic function. Although a possible concern, the likelihood of an acute compartment syndrome was very low in this case.

What would be the next area to examine with this patient?

The therapist in this situation examined the cast to check whether it had been fitted too tightly. Because the patient had a full leg cast, only an attempt could be made to palpate the area around the toes on the dorsal and plantar surfaces of the foot. Noting that the space between the cast and skin was minimal at best, the therapist recommended the physician be informed of the possibility that the cast was too tight. Neurologic symptoms consistent with loss of motor function in the anterior compartment indicated possible increased pressure to the peroneal nerve where it comes over the neck of the fibula.

Diagnosis

Physical Therapist Practice Patterns 4G: Impaired Joint Mobility, Muscle Performance, and Range of Motion Associated with Fracture and 5F: Impaired Peripheral Nerve Integrity and Muscle Performance Associated with Peripheral Nerve Injury.

What was the correct response to the patient's refusal to attempt ambulation?

Intervention

The therapist contacted the physician, who immediately ordered that the cast be windowed laterally to relieve pressure from the peroneal nerve over the neck of the fibula. The physician also requested that she be contacted immediately after the windowing of the cast to be apprised of the sensory and motor aspects of the patient's condition.

Once cast pressure was relieved, the numbness on the dorsum of the foot dissipated, and sensory function was restored. Within 30 minutes, sensory and motor function returned to the toes. Had sensory and motor function not returned quickly, it would have been appropriate to again consider the presence of a compartment syndrome.

Outcome

Later that day, the patient was refitted with a new long-leg cast. He was then able to tolerate crutch training and ambulation. The patient was discharged from the hospital with instructions to keep the extremity elevated and to remain non–weight-bearing for 6 weeks. He experienced no additional motor or sensory problems.

RECOMMENDED READINGS

Bae DS, Kadiyala RK, Waters PM: Acute compartment syndrome in children: contemporary diagnosis, treatment, and outcome, *J Pediatr Orthop* 21:680, 2001.

Bono CM, Levine RG, Rao JP, Behrens FF: Nonarticular proximal tibia fractures: treatment options and decision making, *J Am Acad Orthop Surg* 9:176, 2001.

Mubarak SJ, Hargens AR, Karkal SS: Coping with the diagnostic complexities of the compartment syndrome, *Emerg Med Rep* 9:185, 1998.

Perron AD, Brady WJ, Keats TE: Acute compartment syndrome, *Am J Emerg Med* 19:413, 2001.

LEARNING OBJECTIVES

The reader will be able to:

1. Describe a possible mechanism of injury resulting in a torn quadriceps tendon.

2. List examination strategies to help determine if a quadriceps tendon is torn.

3. Discuss alternative interventions for a patient with a torn quadriceps tendon.

The reader should know that an 80-year-old man with arthritis was referred to physical therapy for postsurgical rehabilitation of a right total knee arthroplasty. The patient arrived at a therapist's office in a wheelchair from home after having been discharged 2 days earlier from a rehabilitation hospital. He required moderate assistance to get out of the car and into the wheelchair. During the transfer, the patient indicated that he had considerable difficulty maintaining knee extension and that he could not place much weight on the extremity without feeling as though it were going to collapse. The patient first noticed he was having problems with weight bearing and keeping the knee straight after attempting a pivot transfer into his car after discharge from the rehabilitation hospital.

The knee exhibited swelling not uncommon for a recent total knee arthroplasty. Active-assisted flexion was 100 degrees, and full extension could be obtained only passively while the patient was in the long sitting position. The patient ambulated with a walker, a knee immobilizer, and with a very short-stride gait. It appeared that he was placing minimal weight on the right lower extremity. He was unable to perform a straight-leg raise and demonstrated a very weak quadriceps contraction that was palpable only in the mid-quadriceps. No significant patellar movement was noted on attempts to actively elicit a quadriceps contraction.

During the next two visits to the clinic, attempts to improve the patient's gait pattern and lessen the extension lag were unsuccessful.

There was decreased flexibility in the hamstring muscles. The patient reported that he was not making progress with his home program.

Examination

HISTORY

The patient was a well-educated man who expressed his opinion that he sustained an injury to the knee at the time of transfer. He indicated he felt a "pop and a sharp pain" at the time he was being assisted from the wheelchair to the car. He indicated that he mentioned the problem to the staff at the rehabilitation center during the transfer. The staff indicated that he should not be concerned.

SYSTEMS REVIEW

The patient had a history of high blood pressure controlled by daily medication. He reported no other significant past medical history. There were no reports of low back pain or discomfort. He reported no plans to have further total joint surgeries because of the difficulties experienced with his first replacement.

TESTS AND MEASURES

Strength in the uninvolved lower extremity was within normal limits. Sensation was intact throughout.

Evaluation

What problem was suspected?

It was surmised that at some point during the transfer into the car at the rehabilitation hospital, the patient sustained a tear of the quadriceps tendon at its insertion. The tear was identified visually and by palpation by requesting the patient to perform a short-arc quadriceps exercise. Although there was virtually no pain while the patient attempted the short arc, very little or no movement could be seen or palpated.

What was the most appropriate next step?

Diagnosis

Physical Therapist Practice Pattern 4H: Impaired Joint Mobility, Motor Function, Muscle Performance, and Range of Motion Associated with Joint Arthroplasty.

Intervention

Upon recommendation of the therapist, the patient was immediately seen by his orthopedic surgeon. The surgeon advised the patient of the torn tendon and indicated that if a repair were to be made, it would have to be performed within the next several days. If not repaired soon, the tendon would retract to the point where reattachment would be difficult or impossible. It was the physician's opinion that rehabilitation would begin after a long period of immobilization. The knee would have to be in full extension for at least 4 weeks.

Outcome

A quadriceps tear is considered rare after total knee arthroplasty. If present, it is usually associated with trauma. When a tear has occurred, repair is best done immediately. After reattachment, the knee frequently must be maintained in full extension for several weeks. Regaining range of motion after these repairs may be difficult. In this instance, the patient decided not to have the repair. He preferred wearing a brace rather than enduring another operation and rehabilitation.

What was the focus of subsequent therapy visits and the home program?

Therapy focused on general conditioning, ambulation, and the use of a knee brace to help control knee flexion. The therapist and patient worked toward the goal of independence in ambulation and activities of daily living in the home environment. After 3 weeks of daily physical therapy, the patient was discharged as independent with the use of a walker.

RECOMMENDED READINGS

Bedor M: Quadriceps protects the anterior cruciate ligament, *J Orthop Res* 19:629, 2001.

Campbell R, Evans M, Tucker M, et al: Why don't patients do their exercises? Understanding non-compliance with physiology in patients with osteoarthritis of the knee, *J Epidemiol Community Health* 55:132, 2001.

Cole BJ, Harner CD: Degenerative arthritis of the knee in active patients: evaluation and management, *J Am Acad Orthop Surg* 7:389, 1999.

Enad JG: Patellar tendon ruptures, *South Med J* 92:563, 1999.

Hansen L, Larsen S, Laulund T: Traumatic bilateral tendon rupture, *J Orthop Sci* 6:187, 2001.

Kelly BM, Rao N, Louis SS, et al: Bilateral, simultaneous, spontaneous rupture of quadriceps tendons without trauma in an obese patient: a case report, *Arch Phys Med Rehabil* 82:415, 2001.

Konrath GA, Chen D, Lock T, et al: Outcomes following repair of quadriceps tendon ruptures, *J Orthop Trauma* 12:273, 1998.

Labib SA, Hage WD: A simple technique for transpatellar fixation of quadriceps tendon rupture, *Orthopedics* 24:743, 2001.

Miller ME, Rejeski WJ, Messier SP, Loeser RF: Modifiers of change in physical functioning in older adults with knee pain: the observational arthritis study in seniors (OASIS), *Arthritis Rheum* 45:331, 2001.

Rejeski WJ, Miller ME, Foy C, et al: Self-efficacy and the progression of functional limitations and self-reported disability in older adults with knee pain, *J Gerontol B Psychol Sci Soc Sci* 56:S261, 2001.

Rougraff BT, Reeck CC, Essenmacher J: Complete quadriceps tendon ruptures, *Orthopedics* 19:509, 1996.

Scranton PE: Management of knee pain and stiffness after total knee arthroplasty, *J Arthroplasty* 16:428, 2001.

Shelbourne KD, Darmelio MP, Klootwyk TE: Patellar tendon rupture repair using Dall-Miles cable, *Am J Knee Surg* 14:17, 2001.

Yilmaz C, Binnet MS, Narman S: Tendon lengthening repair and early mobilization in treatment of neglected bilateral simultaneous traumatic rupture of the quadriceps tendon, *Knee Surg Sports Traumatol Arthrosc* 9:163, 2001.

LEARNING OBJECTIVES

The reader will be able to:

1. Describe how diagnostic testing may influence a physical therapy plan of care.
2. Discuss how a patient's clinical progression may be influenced by a physician's medical choices.

Examination

HISTORY

A 46-year-old female arrived at a physical therapy clinic after sustaining a left proximal humeral fracture. That fracture had occurred 6 weeks earlier when she tripped over a baby stroller and landed on her left arm. The patient had her arm in a sling until 1 week earlier. She was referred for physical therapy by her family physician.

What additional information was needed from this patient's history?

The patient was the primary caretaker for her 1-year-old granddaughter. She was also going to school part time and working part time as a legal aide. The patient was right-hand dominant. She had no significant medical history except intermittent chronic low back pain. The only medication she took was regular-strength Tylenol for shoulder pain, as needed. She rated her pain at rest as a 5 on scale of 0 to 10, and 8 with any movement of the arm.

What tests and measures were appropriate for this patient?

TESTS AND MEASURES

With the patient supine, her left shoulder active range of motion (ROM) was measured as 10 degrees of flexion, extension, and abduction. External and internal rotation could not be measured because of the patient's pain and guarding. Shoulder passive ROM was 30 degrees of flexion, 10 degrees of extension, and 30 degrees of abduction.

Manual muscle testing of the shoulder flexors and abductors produced scores of –2/5. The patient's shoulder end feel in all directions was empty secondary to guarding. No significant swelling was seen, but moderate tenderness was noted on the anterior aspect of the shoulder.

Were there any other important items to address in the examination?

Instrumental activities of daily living were reviewed. The patient had moderate difficulty donning and doffing her shirt.

Diagnosis

Physical Therapist Preferred Practice Pattern 4G: Impaired Joint Mobility, Muscle Performance, and Range of Motion Associated with Fracture.

Prognosis

The prognosis for this patient was judged as fair because she had a moderate loss of function. There were also the complicating but motivating factors of childcare, work, and school. Overall, the patient was in good physical health; therefore, prolonged impairments were initially expected to be minimal to none.

Intervention

The plan of care for this patient included moist heat, passive ROM, active/active-assisted ROM, ice, and a home exercise program. In the first month, the patient showed an increase in shoulder ROM, but no reduction in pain. After the second month, the patient's ROM reached a plateau, and her pain levels increased.

What was an appropriate course of action for the therapist to take?

The physical therapist contacted the family physician and recommended diagnostic imaging (specifically, magnetic resonance imaging [MRI]), because of lack of progression and increase in pain. The physician felt that MRI was not needed, and changed the diagnosis to "frozen shoulder." A request was made to continue with "aggressive physical therapy."

The patient returned to the clinic, where the therapist added aggressive ROM exercises and electrical stimulation to help with pain control. The patient did not tolerate aggressive ROM; therefore, the range was done to her tolerance. After a few sessions, the patient's pain was noted to have increased with no significant increase in ROM.

Finally, after a month, the family physician agreed to order MRI and consultation with an orthopedist. Two weeks later, the patient returned to continue with physical therapy after undergoing a manipulation under anesthesia. A referral slip from the family physician read "continue physical therapy."

What information was appropriate for the therapist to review before resuming intervention?

The physical therapist requested the MRI results, which showed inferior subluxation of the humeral head, a torn glenoid labrum posteriorly, an osseous fragment, and probable partial tear of the supraspinatus and infraspinatus tendons. After reexamination, a call was placed to the family physician regarding the results of the MRI. The physician wanted to continue rehabilitation at the therapist's discretion. The physical therapist then contacted the orthopedist to schedule a follow-up appointment. Subsequently, an arthroscopic surgical repair was performed.

Outcome

The patient returned to physical therapy and regained full functional ROM and strength with intermittent pain. She was discharged from therapy to continue with a home exercise program, and was able to return to work without difficulty.

Discussion

In this case the physical therapist used good professional judgment and facilitated a correct referral. The patient benefited from prompt surgical intervention and follow-up physical therapy intervention.

RECOMMENDED READINGS

Magee DJ: *Orthopedic physical assessment* (ed 3), Philadelphia: WB Saunders, 1997.
Goodman CC, Snyder TE: *Differential diagnosis in physical therapy* (ed 3), Philadelphia: WB Saunders, 2000.
McKinnis LN: *Fundamentals of orthopedic radiology*, Philadelphia: FA Davis, 1997.

LEARNING OBJECTIVES

The reader will be able to:

1. Discuss the physical therapy needs of the patient with multiple trauma.
2. Discuss what clinical factors may need to be considered when recommending electrodiagnostic studies.
3. Describe at what point physical therapy should be discontinued when no progress is made toward set goals or when progress has plateaued.

Examination

HISTORY

A 4-year-old girl was mistakenly run over by her mother while on a riding lawn mower. The patient sustained an open fracture to the right femur, tibia, and multiple bones of the foot. She also had extensive soft tissue, vascular, and nerve damage. She underwent 23 surgeries, including external fixators of the femur, tibia, and fibula; multiple skin grafts; and revascularization by surgically attaching her legs together. The patient presented at a physical therapy clinic at age 5 with her mother.

What other information from the patient's history was needed?

The patient was in kindergarten and lived at home with both parents and four siblings. She was very active, had no other health problems, and liked to do physical activities. She wanted to be able to roller-skate and ice skate. The patient was 6 weeks status post surgery of grafting the wounds from separating the legs and reattachment of the quadriceps tendon.

What tests and measures were appropriate for this patient?

The patient had extensive bound scarring on the entire right anterior leg, with loss of all sensation. She had a full-thickness wound along the incision site on the thigh.

She ambulated with knee-ankle-foot orthosis (KAFO) with a ratchet lock, non–weight-bearing, and used a walker. She had a leg length discrepancy of 1.25 inches and foot length discrepancy of 1 inch on the right. Additionally, according to diagnostic imaging reports, she had no growth plates left in the knee or ankle joints. Her knee was in a flexion contracture of 30 degrees, and manually she demonstrated –25 degrees of full extension. The end feel had some give, but was not hard. At the time, there was trace quadriceps, hamstring, anterior tibialis, and gastrocsoleous muscle activity.

Ankle passive range of motion (ROM) was minimal. The contralateral leg and bilateral upper extremities demonstrated normal strength, ROM, and function.

Diagnosis

This patient's case was very complex, as reflected by the choice of four Physical Therapist Preferred Practice Patterns:

- 4G: Impaired Joint Mobility, Muscle Performance, and Range of Motion Associated with Fracture.
- 4I: Impaired Joint Mobility, Motor Function, Muscle Performance, and Range of Motion Associated with Bony or Soft Tissue Injury.
- 5F: Impaired Peripheral Nerve Integrity and Muscle Performance Associated with Peripheral Nerve Injury.
- 7E: Impaired Integumentary Integrity Associated with Skin Involvement Extending into Fascia, Muscle, or Bone and Scar Formation.

Prognosis

The referring orthopedist believed that the patient's overall prognosis was poor. That physician believed that unless the patient's ROM and quadriceps strength increased, amputation would be necessary.

What would a physical therapy plan of care entail? What factors need to be considered?

Intervention

The patient was seen three times per week for 3 months after school. The patient's mother was always present at the treatment sessions and because she had no childcare, she always brought the patient's 6-year-old sister.

The plan of care included active, active-assisted, and passive ROM exercises; strengthening exercises; gait training; scar mobilization; electric stimulation for muscle reeducation; balance training; and dynamic splinting.

Outcome

After 3 months, the patient was able to ambulate without the KAFO but continued to use a walker, weight bearing as tolerated on the right lower extremity. There was no increase in strength, ROM, or scar mobility. The patient also began to complain of severe pain in her involved leg. The physical therapist contacted the referring physician to inform him of the patient's status. The therapist also discussed the possibility of sending the patient for electrodiagnostic testing (electromyography and nerve conduction studies) to check innervation of the right lower extremity. Those studies demonstrated a lack of innervation of the quadriceps and dorsiflexor muscles. The physical therapy was stopped. Because of intractable pain and poor functional gains, the patient had a knee disarticulation amputation approximately 1 month later.

RECOMMENDED READINGS

Aitken ME, Jaffe KM, DiScala C, Rivara FP: Functional outcome in children with multiple trauma without significant head injury, *Arch Phys Med Rehabil* 80:889, 1999.

National Pediatric Trauma Registry, Research and Training Center on Rehabilitation and Childhood Trauma: The National Pediatric Trauma Registry: Injuries among children, *Pediatr Phys Ther* 7:24, 1995.

Haley SM, Baryza MJ, Webster HC: Pediatric rehabilitation and recovery of children with traumatic injuries, *Pediatr Phys Ther* 4:24, 1992.

Case **43**

LEARNING OBJECTIVES

The reader will be able to:

1. Discuss the clinical signs and symptoms associated with Meniere's disease.

2. Identify and differentiate clinical signs and symptoms associated with medications commonly used to treat Meniere's disease.

3. Discuss what impairments may be permanent and how they might be compensated for.

4. Identify appropriate referral sources for a patient with Meniere's disease.

5. Discuss how to apply the principals of neurological treatment theories in developing intervention strategies for a high-level functioning patient with Meniere's disease.

Background On Diagnosis

Meniere's disease is associated with overproduction of endolymph or fluid in the ears, which affects auditory and vestibular function. Common precipitating factors include viral infections or trauma. Clinical signs and symptoms include reports of transient but severe attacks of dizziness or vertigo that incapacitate the individual. Nausea, vomiting, abnormal eye movement (nystagmus), and sensorineural hearing loss (tinnitus) are also common findings. Acute attacks may last a few minutes to several hours, with residual affects reported weeks to months later. Medical treatment includes the use of central nervous system suppressant, diuretic, or antiemetic medications. Individuals with Meniere's disease are advised to decrease consumption of salt, caffeine, alcohol, and tobacco. Physical therapy has also proven beneficial.[1-3,5]

The reader should know that a 26-year-old female was diagnosed with Meniere's disease after an episode of vertigo. She was originally unable to sit, stand, or walk without episodes of severe nausea and vomiting, which lasted for 10 days. At the time of the initial physical therapy examination, she was able to do all of the above, but reported feeling very unsteady. She reported that she had begun to identify what she referred to as "triggers" for attacks as being repetitive vertical patterns,

moving or flashing lights, unsteady floors (elevators, docks, escalators), or busy floor and wall patterns. She reported that during attacks she noticed things spinning from right to left and she had a tendency to fall to the right when experiencing attacks. She was taking meclizine (Antivert) four times per day and trimethobenzamide (Tigan) as needed to control the vomiting. She also had a history of lupus erythematosus.

Examination

HISTORY

The patient, a 26-year-old single female, reported experiencing a sudden onset of vertigo after an intense aerobic workout 4 months earlier. She was treated and released from the emergency room with intravenous fluids, meclizine, and antibiotics for a possible ear infection. The symptoms persisted off and on for approximately 2 weeks but did not interfere with her normal activities. She experienced a second attack approximately 6 weeks later while at work. She saw her family physician and received a new prescription of meclizine. The symptoms lasted for approximately 2 weeks, and she again was able to resume all normal activities.

When the most recent attack occurred, the patient decided to follow up with her family physician and a neurologist. The symptoms had persisted for more than 2 weeks, and she

177

was not able to work or function even around the house for more than a few minutes. Magnetic resonance imaging of the head revealed inflammation around the eighth cranial nerve. Blood work showed slightly elevated sedimentation rates, but no different than her previous levels. The patient saw a neurologist, who offered options of surgical rhizotomy, continuing medication therapy, and a trial of physical therapy.

The patient reported a history of systemic lupus erythematosus, which was managed through diet and exercise. She reported her main symptoms from the lupus as fluctuating weight, facial and upper torso skin rash, and periodic joint and muscle pain and weakness. Before the recent attacks she had been active, playing field hockey 2 or 3 days per week for a competitive club team and lifting weights and running 4 or 5 days per week. Since the attack, she was happy to be able to stand and walk for short distances. She reported she was able to sit for 15 to 20 minutes and stand and walk for 5 to 10 minutes before symptoms increased to the point at which she would need to lie down. She was not able to work, drive, or use the telephone on the right side. She reported the medication was causing blurred vision, and consequently she had difficulty reading. She had noticed that if she could find external focal points, she could usually keep attacks from becoming full blown, although admitted she was not always successful and still experienced two or three bouts of nausea and vomiting a day. She also said that she was walking much more slowly than normal and preferred to stay close to walls or railings when possible.

The patient was employed as an outpatient physical therapist in a very busy clinic, but had been on sick leave and using vacation time since the most recent attack. She lived in a third-floor apartment with her sister and was relying on friends and family to transport her to appointments.

SYSTEMS REVIEW

Integumentary system. Discoid lesions were noted on the patient's face and upper torso consistent in appearance to those commonly associated with lupus erythematosus. Otherwise, the integumentary system was intact.

Cardiopulmonary system. The patient's cardiopulmonary system was intact.

Musculoskeletal system. The patient's musculoskeletal system was intact, with no visible atrophy or edema at time of initial examination.

Neuromuscular system. The neuromuscular system was the main focus of examination.

TESTS AND MEASURES

The following test results were obtained:
- Loss of gaze stability with the head thrust test as described previously.[2]
- Positive Romberg's test: able to stand for 10 seconds with eyes open; immediate loss of balance with eyes closed.[1,2]
- Positive single-leg stance: immediate loss of balance with eyes open, not attempted with eyes closed.[1]

Gait disturbance was noted, with decreased step and stride length, decreased speed, wide base of support and no trunk rotation or arm swing. The patient was constantly reaching for objects to steady herself and was unable to turn her head while walking without loss of balance. Transfers were independent but slow, and the patient needed to pause for 1 to 2 minutes for dizziness and nausea to pass and for gaze to stabilize.

Evaluation

Based on the initial examination findings, which impairments are temporary and can be remedied?

How much improvement can be expected and how soon will it occur?

The patient's problems (functional limitations and impairments) were characterized as follows:
- Unable to sit for more than 15 to 20 minutes.
- Unable to stand for more than 5 to 10 minutes.
- Ambulation unstable.

- Unable to drive.
- Unable to use telephone on right side.
- Unable to work.
- Unable to work out or participate in social activities.

Diagnosis

Physical Therapist Preferred Practice Pattern 5F: Impaired Peripheral Nerve Integrity and Muscle Performance Associated with Peripheral Nerve Injury.

Prognosis

Over the course of 4 to 8 months, the patient should demonstrate optimal peripheral nerve integrity and muscle performance and the highest level of functioning in home, work (job/school/play), community, and leisure environments, within the context of the impairments, functional limitations, and disabilities. The expected number of visits is between 12 and 56.[4]

GOALS

The long-term (2 months) goals for this patient were to return to normal work, social, and recreational activities. The short-term (1 to 2 weeks) goals included independent sitting, standing, and ambulation for 300 feet to return to normal work, social, recreational, and therapeutic activities.

Interventions

Gaze-retraining exercises were used to help reestablish positional sense. Exercises were performed in a variety of positions (e.g., supine, prone, semirecumbent) with head position changes, as the patient was able to progress.[1-3,5]

Exercises and activities were used to promote habituation. This was accomplished through repeated exposure to noxious stimuli as identified by the patient. As the patient regained control of her ability to focus more rapidly, modifications were made to the environment, including altering the surface on which she was located and increasing the number of distractors within the environment.[1-3,5]

Balance-retraining activities were also included in the program. Besides the Romberg, tandem Romberg, and single-leg stance activities, these included such activities as riding on an elevator with eyes open and eyes closed, sitting or laying on a physioball with eyes open and eyes closed, and sitting on a rolling stool and moving the stool in all directions and rotating in both directions.[1-3,5]

Might this patient have benefited from any other services?

The patient was referred to an otolaryngologist and an audiologist for the hearing deficits and reports of tinnitus.

Which impairments are permanent and must be compensated for?

Outcome

After completing 8 weeks of three times per week outpatient therapy, the patient reported experiencing only two attacks in the preceding month. She was able to regain her sense of equilibrium within a minute or two both times. She had returned to work full time and was able to drive without difficulty. She was still experiencing dizziness when riding elevators or escalators, but had been practicing with eyes open and closed when able. She had resumed running 1 to 2 miles three to four times a week and weightlifting three times a week. She had not yet resumed playing field hockey, because she still felt unsteady if she repeatedly bent forward and stood up. She also reported no longer even attempting to use the telephone on her right side because of the persistent tinnitus. She reported difficulty riding a jet ski, in that she kept tipping over to the right and thought the equipment was faulty, but then she realized that this was a higher-level skill that she had not yet mastered. She also reported reluctance to attempt to ride roller coasters because of the quick directional changes.

She was scheduled to have her hearing tested every 6 months.

If this patient were to return to physical therapy at this stage, what type of activities would likely be included in the intervention?

The activities described as difficult, aside from the use of a telephone, all appeared to require the ability to balance without the normal proprioceptive input from the lower extremities while weight bearing. During all of the above activities the patient was exposed to quick changes in direction and required to stabilize in multiple planes simultaneously. The patient would also be exposed to rapidly changing visual input. This patient did return for a short course of physical therapy (eight visits), during which aquatic therapy activities were used to simulate the multiplanar forces encountered in such activities. Various flotation devices were used along with manual perturbations and water turbulence to increase or decrease the intensity of the balance activities. Activities were performed first with eyes open and later with eyes closed. After the short course of therapy, the patient had again resumed riding roller coasters and jet skis, and playing field hockey. She also reported feeling more steady when riding elevators or escalators.

REFERENCES

1. Goodman CC, Boissonnault WG: *Pathology implications for the physical therapist,* Philadelphia: WB Saunders, 1998.
2. O'Sullivan SB, Schmitz TJ: *Physical rehabilitation assessment and treatment* (ed 4), Philadelphia: FA Davis, 2001.
3. Umphred DA: *Neurological rehabilitation* (ed 4), Philadelphia: Mosby, 2001.
4. American Physical Therapy Association: Guide to physical therapist practice, second edition, *Phys Ther* 81:9, 2001.
5. Gonzalez EG, Meyers SJ, Edelstein JE, et al: *Downey and Darling's physiological basis of rehabilitation medicine* (ed 3), Boston: Butterworth Heinemann, 2001.

LEARNING OBJECTIVES

The reader will be able to:

1. Discuss indications for a molded ankle-foot orthosis and for its reimbursement.
2. Describe basic principles of the prospective payment system (PPS) in skilled nursing facilities.
3. Differentiate PPS and Medicare Part B.
4. Identify the modifications needed in a physical therapy plan of care for a patient living in a retirement community.

The reader should know that an 81-year-old female with degenerative joint disease of the right knee underwent a total knee arthroplasty. Six days after her surgery, she was placed in a skilled nursing facility (SNF) for rehabilitation before returning to her apartment, where she lived alone. Her apartment was part of an independent-living retirement community. She was used to an independent lifestyle in her apartment, but in the SNF she received 24-hour nursing care. The apartment was on one floor, had wall-to-wall carpeting except for tiled floors in the kitchen and bathroom, and a full-sized bathtub. She needed to demonstrate the ability to independently perform all activities of daily living before returning to her apartment. There was full handicap access throughout the community, and all meals were provided (although there was a kitchen in each unit if the residents desired to cook). The housekeeping department also cleaned all bathrooms weekly, but the residents were responsible for their own laundry and general upkeep of the rest of their apartment. The patient had 94 PPS days remaining.

Examination

HISTORY

The patient's past medical history was significant for type 1 diabetes with mild distal lower extremity neuropathies (affecting only sensation on the distal dorsal and plantar surfaces of her feet), and a left total knee arthroplasty done 2 years earlier.

SYSTEMS REVIEW

The patient presented with no history of cardiac or pulmonary problems. Seated/resting vital signs were heart rate, 72 beats per minute; blood pressure, 116/76 mm Hg; and respirations, 18 breaths per minute. She was allowed weight bearing as tolerated through the right lower extremity. She was unable to tolerate narcotics for pain control because they made her nauseous. She received insulin injections to control her diabetes.

TESTS AND MEASURES

On examination, active range of motion (ROM) of the right knee was −16 degrees extension and 30 degrees flexion. Passive ROM of the right knee was −13 degrees extension and 75 degrees flexion. Strength of the right knee was 3−/5 for flexion and extension.

The patient experienced a right foot drop postoperatively and had been provided with an off-the-shelf molded ankle-foot orthosis (MAFO) by the acute-care hospital. Her right ankle dorsiflexors presented as flaccid, and sensation to light touch, pinprick, and temperature were diminished on the anterior and lateral surfaces of the right lower leg and dorsal right foot. Skin inspection of the lower extremities was unremarkable except for a 9-inch clean incision on the right knee that was healing well.

Midpatellar girth measurements of the right and left knees were 49 and 42.8 cm, respectively. Pain levels were 8 out of 10 with ROM and 10 out of 10 with weight bearing on

the affected leg. All transfers were performed with minimal assistance of one, and
the patient ambulated 15 feet with a standard
walker and minimal assistance of one. She
complained of severe discomfort with the
MAFO, and on closer examination, it was
determined that her heel was too wide for it.
The MAFO was also causing her to invert
and plantar-flex her right foot whenever she
bore weight through the right lower extremity.

Diagnosis

Physical Therapist Practice Pattern 4H:
Impaired Joint Mobility, Motor Function,
Muscle Performance, and Range of Motion
Associated with Joint Arthroplasty.

Evaluation

*How could the positioning of her right
foot in the off-the-shelf MAFO affect
the right knee?*

It was never determined exactly, per the orthopedic surgeon, why this patient developed a
right foot drop. The inclination was that after
the leg became edematous postoperatively,
the increased pressure around the knee
compromised the common peroneal nerve.
Unfortunately, no follow-up testing was performed to make an exact determination.

The acute-care hospital staff gave the
patient the off-the-shelf MAFO versus a
custom-fitted one because they believed that
the foot drop would resolve rather quickly.
They also did not correlate the increased knee
pain with the ill-fitting MAFO. Her inverted
and plantar-flexed foot was causing a significant increase in varus force at the right knee,
which appeared to be the chief cause of the
increased pain. She was able to ambulate
safely without the MAFO but demonstrated a
severe steppage gait because of the right foot
drop. This was causing her excessive right
knee flexion during the swing phase of
gait, which resulted in increased pain and
swelling, delaying healing. Therefore, to
avoid causing a chronic inflammation in her
knee, it was decided to consult an orthotist

to fabricate a custom-fitted MAFO for the
patient's right foot.

*What were some of the indications and
concerns surrounding a custom-fitted MAFO
for this patient?*

Despite the diagnosis of diabetes (along with
peripheral neuropathy causing altered sensation), the patient was determined to be reliable
to examine her foot after wearing the off-the-
shelf orthosis for signs of skin breakdown.
As opposed to the first orthosis, the custom-
fabricated MAFO normalized forces and
stresses transferring through the foot and
ankle, decreasing the risk of skin ulceration.
The new MAFO also allowed the patient to
assume a more normal gait pattern. Her pain
decreased to 5 out of 10 within 2 days, and
the edema decreased by 3 cm within a week.
In turn, active and passive ROM improved.
Because pressure around the knee was reduced,
nerve recovery could begin, as evidenced by
the return of sensation and trace contractions
in the right dorsiflexors.

*How was the MAFO reimbursed and how
did the PPS apply?*

Medicare is divided into two separate systems
to provide coverage to those who qualify to
receive its benefits. Part A (also known as
PPS) is the hospital and subacute coverage,
which can last for up to 100 days. The require-
ment for a patient to continue coverage as a
Part A is the classification as "skilled." This
means that the patient receives a service that
is performed under the supervision of skilled
nursing or rehabilitation personnel. Skilled
nursing must be provided daily 7 days a week;
therapy services must be provided 5 days per
week. There are also nursing issues that can
"skill" a resident who does not receive rehabilitation services. Examples include patients
with open wounds, intravenous treatments,
insulin-dependent diabetics, feeding tubes,
dialysis, chemotherapy, and a myriad of
other reasons. However, depending on the
complexity of these nursing issues, the
amount of reimbursement can vary.

Because the patient was an admission under the Medicare Part A (or PPS), the MAFO was not directly reimbursed by Medicare. The regulations required that the SNF provide equipment and supplies for patients as needed, and the funding for those supplies came out of the money prospectively paid by Medicare. This means that the SNF received the same funding regardless whether the MAFO was purchased. It was then an expense from the facility's budget, not Medicare's budget.

Part B is considered Medicare's outpatient insurance, though someone living in a skilled nursing facility can receive Part B services if he or she does not qualify for Part A. Part B is a more traditional fee-for-services system and covers 80% of the services provided. The remaining 20% is covered by a secondary insurance, or must be privately paid. There is no set number of days or minutes that must be achieved to qualify for reimbursement, though the Centers for Medicare and Medicaid Services has its own fee schedule for treatments, modalities, etc. (i.e. currently $65 for a physical therapy evaluation). Part B will pay for 80% of most durable medical equipment, and also orthotics and prosthetics. Therefore, with this case, the patient had Part A benefits and the MAFO's cost had to be subtracted out of the prospective payment. However, under Part B, the MAFO would have been 80% directly reimbursed and at no cost to the facility.

Intervention/Outcome

Occupational therapy's main goal with this patient revolved around lower extremity dressing, because she found this task most difficult. Their treatment sessions incorporated donning and doffing the MAFO, allowing physical therapy to focus on gait, transfers, strengthening, ROM and edema reduction. Also, occupational therapy purchased a tub bench for the patient's bathroom and worked with her to increase safety with homemaking skills. Four weeks after admission, the patient was able to return to her apartment and previous lifestyle.

RECOMMENDED READINGS

Atherly A: Supplemental insurance: Medicare's accidental stepchild, *Med Care Res Rev* 58:131, 2001.

Federal Register 58:60789, 1993.

Gardner J: Groups support PPS for skilled-nursing care, *Mod Healthcare* 25:38, 1995.

Green MF, Aliabadi Z, Green BT: Diabetic foot: evaluation and management, *South Med J* 95:95, 2002.

Papagelopoulos PJ, Sim FH: Limited range of motion after total knee arthroplasty: etiology, treatment, and prognosis, *Orthopedics* 20:1061, 1997.

Vance TN: *Medicare guidelines explained for the physical therapist: a practical guide for physical therapy service delivery*, Reston, Va: St. Anthony's Publishing, 1998.

Case 45

LEARNING OBJECTIVES

The reader will be able to:

1. List forms of diagnostic imaging used to identify deep vein thrombosis and pulmonary embolus.

2. Describe signs and symptoms of a pulmonary embolism.

Examination

HISTORY

The patient, a 72-year-old retired female, was admitted to an acute care hospital through the emergency room with left-sided weakness, headache, and nausea. She was diagnosed with evolving left cerebral vascular accident (CVA) and was immediately placed on an antithrombolytic TPA (tissue plasminogen activator) drug.

During the course of her acute-care stay, she developed warmth, pain, and swelling in her right calf. Homan's sign was positive. Doppler scan was positive for deep vein thrombosis (DVT). She was placed on bed rest for 3 days, with intravenous heparin followed by oral administration of coumadin and TEDS to be worn at all times when allowed out of bed. After an acute care stay of 3 weeks, the patient was transferred to a rehabilitation facility.

On admission to the rehabilitation facility, the patient was 5 feet 2 inches tall and weighed 200 pounds. She reported a sedentary lifestyle, with hobbies of knitting and doing crossword puzzles. She was of Polish descent and liked to prepare and eat ethnic specialty foods, such as kielbasi, pierogies, and potato pancakes. She had smoked for 40 years but quit 10 years earlier secondary to problems with asthma. She resided in a two-story house that had 12 stairs with two railings between the first and second floors and three stairs with two railings to enter the home from outside. She lived with her husband of 50 years and before admission was independent in all activities of daily living (ADL) and instrumental ADLs.

The patient's past medical history included hypertension, diabetes mellitus (adult onset), asthma, degenerative joint disease, cholesterolemia (excessive amounts of cholesterol in the blood), and osteoporosis with a history of compression fracture of T8.

Her medications included lisinopril (Zestril) 20 mg twice a day for hypertension, glyburide (DiaBeta) 5 mg four times a day for diabetes, albuterol (Proventil) 2 puffs twice a day for asthma, celecoxib (Celebrex) 20 mg/day for degenerative joint disease, and atorvastatin (Lipitor) 10 mg/day for cholesterolemia.

REVIEW OF SYSTEMS

- Vital signs: Blood pressure 130/84 mm Hg, heart rate 76 beats per minute (bpm), respirations 18 breaths per minute
- Range of motion/joint mobility: Flaccid right upper extremity, spastic right lower extremity
- Gait, locomotion, balance: Bed mobility, moderate assistance of 1 to roll right to left; transfers, supine → sit moderate assistance of 1; sit ⇔ stand, maximum assistance of 1; stand → pivot maximum assistance of 1; gait, nonambulatory at the time
- Reflexes: Positive Babinski's sign and clonus in the right lower extremity
- Balance: Sitting balance unsupported fair minus
- Endurance: Fair
- Communication: Global aphasia

TESTS AND MEASUREMENTS

Magnetic resonance imaging was positive for a left CVA, and a Doppler study was positive for a previous DVT, now resolved.

Evaluation

What are the possible areas of occlusion that may have lead to this patient's symptoms?

Lesions are most often large, involving the perisylvian area of the frontal, temporal, and parietal lobes. An occlusion of the internal carotid area or the middle cerebral artery at its origin was the most common location. With this particular patient, injury had occurred on the left side of the brain. The frontal lobe of the brain is the site of Broca's area, which provides the motor aspects of speech. The temporal/parietal region is the area that houses the sensory aspects of speech (perception and interpretation of language) known as *Wernicke's area.*

The patient was alert and oriented to person and place but demonstrated difficulty with time accuracy. She presented with global aphasia, allowing her to respond to yes/no questions correctly approximately 40% of the time.

What are the characteristics of global aphasia?

Global aphasia is the most common and most severe form of aphasia. It is characterized by spontaneous speech that is either absent or reduced to a few stereotyped words or sounds. Comprehension is reduced or absent. Repetition, reading, and writing are impaired to the same level as spontaneous speech.

Examination findings were consistent with left CVA. Impairments included tone abnormalities, decreased endurance, decreased cognitive and communication skills, decreased balance, and decreased functional mobility.

Diagnosis

Physical Therapist Practice Pattern 5D: Impaired Motor Function and Sensory Integrity Associated with Nonprogressive Disorders of the Central Nervous System—Acquired in Adolescence or Adulthood.

Prognosis

The patient will achieve optimal function within 12 months, with expected discharge in 3 to 4 weeks.

Intervention

This patient was treated by a multidisciplinary approach comprising speech therapy, to address communication and comprehension; occupational therapy, for training in ADL and self-care activities; and physical therapy, including activities to improve balance, coordination, postural stability, and strength and endurance, including gait training, general mobility, and neuromuscular reeducation.

One week after admission to the rehabilitation facility, while lying on the mat table, the patient began to exhibit signs of anxiety, including rapid breathing, sweating, and rapid extraneous hand movements including holding her chest. She was unable to verbalize her complaints and her response to yes/no questions was more inconsistent than usual. Vital signs were measured and found to be blood pressure, 100/50 mm Hg; heart rate, 100 bpm and weak; and respirations 24 per minute and labored.

What could be the cause of this behavior and how should a therapist respond given the patient's past medical history of DVT, CVA, osteoporosis, and compression fracture?

There could be numerous explanations for this type of behavior. Because this patient had been pleasant and cooperative in the past and never exhibited this type of behavior before, it was reasonable to assume that some type of physical event was contributing to her actions. Although she was unable to verbally express her symptoms, her hand motions appeared to indicate chest discomfort. She had a rapid and weak pulse, low blood pressure, dyspnea, and sweating, all of which can be indicators of pulmonary embolism.

Pulmonary embolism can be a life-threatening condition that can lead to death if not treated immediately. It is typically the result of a venous thrombus that occludes a pulmonary artery. Factors that contribute to increased risk of venous thrombosis also contribute to the risk of pulmonary embolism. These factors include prolonged bed rest or immobilization, especially with concomitant limb paralysis and obesity. Although physical therapists are trained to monitor for DVT in postsurgical and immobile patients, many patients will not have physical complaints or obvious clinical signs. It is important not only to be aware of symptoms of DVT (i.e., edema, dull achiness, color/temperature changes of the extremity, pain, warmth, redness, especially in the calf), but also to stay alert for signs of pulmonary embolus (PE), including sudden anxiety or restlessness, rapid and shallow respirations, tachycardia, chest pain, diaphoresis, and cyanosis. Such changes in a patient's presentation should be reported to a physician immediately.

What diagnostic imaging studies can identify DVT or PE?

To identify a DVT, the gold standard is lower limb venography (a contrast medium is injected and radiographs taken to visualize the veins). This procedure is used to help rule out a DVT. Another technique is venous ultrasound with or without Doppler waveform analysis. Pulmonary angiography or lung perfusion imaging (requiring a radiopharmaceutical injection and a camera to obtain lung images) are often used to detect PE.

What is the standard treatment for DVT or PE?

Treatment usually includes thrombolytic agents. Physical therapy management is important when the patient is again stable and the threat of further emboli is resolved.

Treatment can then include deep-breathing exercises, positioning, and mobilization with progressive activity to improve cardiopulmonary function.

Outcome

Because this was a behavior uncharacteristic of this patient and her motions and vital signs indicated some type of a cardiopulmonary event, the nursing staff and physician were immediately notified. The patient's symptoms appeared to indicate the need for immediate medical attention. This patient was transferred immediately to her wheelchair and escorted by professional personnel (physical therapist/nurse) back to her nursing unit. She was readmitted to the acute-care facility and treated for a PE. Following recovery from the PE, this patient was brought back to the rehabilitation center to finish her rehabilitation. She was discharged from that facility 1 month later to her home with family support.

RECOMMENDED READINGS

American College of Radiology: Appropriateness criteria, 1999, available at http:www.acr.org.

Bruckner M: Circulatory system. In Ballinger P, Frank E (eds): *Merrill's atlas of radiographic positions and radiologic procedures*, St Louis: Mosby, 1999.

Maxey L, Magnusson J: *Rehabilitation of the postsurgical orthopedic patient*, St Louis: Mosby, 2001.

Nunnelee J: Minimize the risk of DVT, *RN* December 1995; 28, 1995.

Rothstein JM, Roy SH, Wolf SL: Communication disorder. In Rothstein JM (ed): *The rehabilitation specialist handbook*, Philadelphia: FA Davis, 1998.

Tortorici M, Apfel P: *Pulmonary angiography: advanced radiographic and angiographic procedures*, Philadelphia: FA Davis 1995.

Watchie J: *Cardiopulmonary physical therapy*, Philadelphia: WB Saunders, 1995.

LEARNING OBJECTIVES

The reader will be able to:

1. Discuss the reasons for performing a physical examination on a homebound patient even though she had been examined in the hospital emergency room.

2. Identify the need for diagnostic imaging in a patient who has already had roentgenograph examination.

3. Discuss the importance of corroborating clinical findings with medical documentation.

The reader should know that an 80-year-old female was referred by her family physician to a home health agency for physical therapy. The patient experienced multiple falls and was having increased difficulty maintaining her independence in her home. Her most recent fall occurred 6 weeks earlier and necessitated her relocation into a new apartment 1 week earlier.

Examination

HISTORY

The patient presented with a complex medical history including a left hip fracture 13 months earlier and a right total hip replacement 7 years earlier. She also had a history of myocardial infarction, degenerative joint disease (especially in the weight-bearing joints of the lower extremities), osteoporosis with compression fractures, dorsal kyphosis, and intermittent swelling in both lower extremities. Additionally, she had a congenital short left foot.

SYSTEMS REVIEW

Vision, hearing, and communication skills were all normal. Pulse was steady at 72 beats per minute at rest.

Upper extremity range of motion (ROM) was essentially within functional limits bilaterally. Left lower extremity ROM was also within functional limits but was longer by approximately 3 cm. The right lower extremity presented with severe pain, which increased with attempts to move. The right knee was restricted to 30 degrees of flexion, and exten-

sion lacked 10 degrees. The right hip was also painful with limitations in motion of 80 degrees flexion, 0 degrees extension, and 25 degrees abduction.

Assessing strength was difficult because of the patient's pain, especially in the lower extremities. On a manual muscle test, strength was estimated as 3–/5 in the right lower extremity and 3+/5 in the upper extremities.

The patient exhibited decreased sensation to light touch in the lower extremities bilaterally. Her balance was fair with the use of a walker and poor without the use of a walker. She was independent with bed mobility, although she did have moderate difficulty as a result of her pain. She ambulated with an unsafe hop-to gait with both lower extremities. Because of her pain and poor endurance, she was able to ambulate only 10 feet. She presented with independent wheelchair mobility.

TESTS AND MEASURES

Right knee ligamentous testing for the medial collateral and lateral collateral ligaments as well as the anterior drawer sign was painful and lax.

Evaluation

The patient was now in a new apartment and highly motivated to remain independent. She appeared to have good potential for rehabilitation with goals to improve the distance of ambulation, decrease her pain and improve the overall safety of her mobility.

Diagnosis

Physical Therapist Practice Patterns 5A: Primary Prevention/Risk Reduction for Loss of Balance and Falling; 4D: Impaired Joint Mobility, Motor Function, Muscle Performance, and Range of Motion Associated with Connective Tissue Dysfunction; and 4B: Impaired Posture.

Intervention

A comprehensive home treatment program was started that involved therapeutic exercises for improving her ROM and strength, and therapeutic activities to improve her balance, safety of ambulation, and overall tolerance for exertion.

After approximately 4 weeks of home physical therapy, she was referred to a local medical center for orthopedic assessment of her continuing right lower extremity pain. Her former orthopedist suggested that she may have had a loosening of the right hip prosthesis. There was no orthopedic decision concerning her right hip, but the knee diagnosis was bursitis, which was treated with a cortisone injection.

The patient made excellent progress over the next 5 weeks of intervention in her home. Her ambulation improved so that she was able to walk with one hand assist and with a minimal limp. She could also ascend and descend one flight of steps with two handrails and minimal assistance. Her ambulatory endurance was approximately 15 meters. Her right knee flexion had improved to 90 degrees without pain. Plans were being made to discharge the patient from physical therapy care to a home exercise program.

However, while the treating therapist was away, the patient was sitting outside in her wheelchair when a strong gust of wind blew her over backward and she fell out of her wheelchair and off of a curb. This occurred even though the wheelchair was locked. She was evaluated at the hospital's Emergency Room. Radiographs were negative. She was returned to her home.

The treating therapist was scheduled for a vacation; therefore, a colleague was the first physical therapist to see the patient after the fall from the wheelchair. The colleague's report indicated that the patient felt pain from her right buttock to her toes when attempting to move her right lower extremity. Her pain limited accurate ROM measurements but she was limited to approximately 10 degrees internal rotation and 15 degrees external rotation, and other hip and knee motions were essentially within functional limits. She was able to stand up independently but used a toe-touch to partial weight-bearing gait for only 10 feet with the use of her walker. Because of pain, the patient's mobility and exercise were markedly limited.

The emergency room diagnosis after radiographs was deep muscle bruising. What else could have been considered?

Six days after the most recent fall, the treating physical therapist returned for continued home physical therapy. The discharge papers from the emergency room were reviewed and indicated no fracture. However, the patient complained of severe pain that she rated at a 10 on a 0 to 10 pain scale, with marked limitation in right ankle ROM at –10 degrees dorsiflexion, 30 degrees plantarflexion, 5 degrees inversion, and 10 degrees eversion. Swelling was present in the lateral ankle, and moderate to severe tenderness was noted over the lateral malleolus and distal fibula. The strength of plantarflexion, inversion, and eversion were all scored as 1/5. Ambulation was a hop-to gait using a walker.

What course of action could be taken?

Outcome

The clinical findings suggested that the patient may have sustained an injury to the right ankle. The inability to bear weight in connection with the swelling, tenderness, and pain were all indicative of a possible fracture.

The therapist contacted the home health agency to report the foregoing findings. Also, the emergency room records were reviewed to confirm the exact site that had been radiographed at the time of the fall. The emergency room discharge papers did not indicate which body part or parts had been examined. Until the possible injury to the involved ankle was clarified, no further weight bearing, ROM, or strengthening exercises were attempted for the lower extremities.

Discussion

After communication with the hospital's radiology department, it was learned that only the hip and knee were radiographed in the emergency room. The coordinator of home health services for the home health agency communicated that information to the family physician, who ordered a radiograph of the ankle. A courtesy telephone call had already been placed to the referring orthopedic physician. The new radiographs revealed a fracture of the fibula with displacement of the distal fragment.

Physical therapy was continued in the home. At the request of the family physician, the patient was given a knee immobilizer for the right fibular fracture and an elastic wrap to reduce swelling. When the elastic wrap was removed, the skin was damp and remained compressed for more than 40 minutes. Again, contact was made with the home health agency to coordinate care.

Finally, 1 week after the fracture, the patient was seen by an orthopedist, who put an air cast on the fracture site and approved ambulation with a walker.

RECOMMENDED READINGS

Brimer M, Moran M: *Clinical cases in physical therapy*, Boston: Butterworth-Heinemann, 1995.

American Physical Therapy Association: Guide to physical therapist practice, second edition, *Phys Ther* 81:1, 2001.

Kauffman T: *Geriatric rehabilitation manual*, Philadelphia: Churchill Livingstone, 1999.

McRae R: *Practical fracture treatment* (ed 3), Philadelphia: Churchill Livingstone, 1994.

Appendix

CASE PRACTICE PATTERN DESIGNATION AND CASE COMPLEXITY—LOWEST TO HIGHEST

Addressing Issues or Information Outside Designated Practice Pattern(s).
Cases: 24, 1, 3

Practice Pattern 4A: Primary Prevention/Risk Reduction for Skeletal Demineralization.
Case: 6

Practice Pattern 4B: Impaired Posture
Cases: 46, 6

Practice Pattern 4D: Impaired Joint Mobility, Motor Function, Muscle Performance, and Range of Motion Associated with Connective Tissue Dysfunction.
Cases: 29, 46, 22, 2, 27, 18

Practice Pattern 4E: Impaired Joint Mobility, Motor Function, Muscle Performance, and Range of Motion Associated with Localized Inflammation.
Cases: 35, 11, 19, 9

Practice Pattern 4F: Impaired Joint Mobility, Motor Function, Muscle Performance, Range of Motion, and Reflex Integrity Associated with Spinal Disorders.
Cases: 29, 23

Practice Pattern 4G: Impaired Joint Mobility, Muscle Performance, and Range of Motion Associated with Fracture.
Cases: 39, 41, 42

Practice Pattern 4H: Impaired Joint Mobility, Motor Function, Muscle Performance, and Range of Motion Associated with Joint Arthroplasty.
Cases: 38, 40, 44

Practice Pattern 4I: Impaired Joint Mobility, Motor Function, Muscle Performance, and Range of Motion Associated with Bony or Soft Tissue Surgery.
Cases: 33, 42, 32, 20

Practice Pattern 4J: Impaired Motor Function, Muscle Performance, Range of Motion, Gait, Locomotion, and Balance Associated with Amputation.
Case: 26

Practice Pattern 5A: Primary Prevention/Risk Reduction for Loss of Balance and Falling.
Cases: 46, 7, 17, 13

Practice Pattern 5B: Impaired Neuromotor Development.
Case: 28

Practice Pattern 5C: Impaired Motor Function and Sensory Integrity Associated with Nonprogressive Disorders of the Central Nervous System—Congenital Origin or Acquired in Infancy or Childhood.
Cases: 4, 37, 12, 26

Practice Pattern 5D: Impaired Motor Function and Sensory Integrity Associated with Nonprogressive Disorders of the Central Nervous System—Acquired in Adolescence or Adulthood.

Cases: 8, 45, 27

Practice Pattern 5E: Impaired Motor Function and Sensory Integrity Associated with Progressive Disorders of the Central Nervous System.

Case: 7

Practice Pattern 5F: Impaired Peripheral Nerve Integrity and Muscle Performance Associated with Peripheral Nerve Injury.

Cases: 39, 42, 21, 23, 43

Practice Pattern 5H: Impaired Motor Function, Peripheral Nerve Integrity, and Sensory Integrity Associated with Nonprogressive Disorders of the Spinal Cord.

Cases: 16, 15, 5, 14

Practice Pattern 6C: Impaired Ventilation, Respiration/Gas Exchange, and Aerobic Capacity/Endurance Associated with Airway Clearance Dysfunction.

Case: 31

Practice Pattern 6D: Impaired Aerobic Capacity/Endurance Associated with Cardiovascular Pump Dysfunction or Failure.

Case: 25

Practice Pattern 7C: Impaired Integumentary Integrity Associated with Partial-Thickness Skin Involvement and Scar Formation.

Case: 30

Practice Pattern 7D: Impaired Integumentary Integrity Associated with Full-Thickness Skin Involvement and Scar Formation.

Cases: 34, 36

Practice Pattern 7E: Impaired Integumentary Integrity Associated with Skin Involvement Extending into Fascia, Muscle, or Bone and Scar Formation.

Case: 42

Guide to Practice: Procedural Interventions, Page s108: Functional Training in Work (job/school/play), Community, and Leisure Integration or Reintegration (including instrumental activities of daily living, work hardening, and work conditioning).

Case: 10

REFERENCES

American Physical Therapy Association: Guide to physical therapist practice, second edition, *Phys Ther* 81:1, 2001.

Index